NT

D0270239

TTC

First published in 2008 by
Liberties Press
Guinness Enterprise Centre | Taylor's Lane | Dublin 8
Tel: +353 (1) 415 1224
www.LibertiesPress.com | info@libertiespress.com

Distributed in the United States by
Dufour Editions | PO Box 7 | Chester Springs | Pennsylvania | 19425

and in Australia by
James Bennett Pty Limited | InBooks | 3 Narabang Way
Belrose NSW 2085

Trade enquiries to CMD Distribution
55A Spruce Avenue | Stillorgan Industrial Park
Blackrock | County Dublin
Tel: +353 (1) 294 2560 | Fax: +353 (1) 294 2564

Copyright © Fiona McPhillips, 2008

The author has asserted her moral rights.

ISBN: 978–1–905483–36–5
2 4 6 8 10 9 7 5 3 1

A CIP record for this title is available from the British Library.

Cover design by Dermot Hall
Illustrations by John Braine
Internal design by Liberties Press
Printed by ScandBook, Sweden

This book is sold subject to the condition that it shall not, by way of trade or otherwise, be lent, resold, hired out or otherwise circulated, without the publisher's prior consent, in any form other than that in which it is published and without a similar condition including this condition being imposed on the subsequent publisher. No part of this publication may be reproduced or transmitted in any form or by any means, electronic or mechanical, including photocopying, recording or storage in any information or retrieval system, without the prior permission of the publisher in writing.

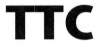

TTC

Trying to Conceive
The Irish Couple's Guide

Fiona McPhillips

For John, James, Anna and the ones that didn't make it

Contents

Foreword

It is ironic that some women spend their twenties worrying about getting pregnant unintentionally, only to find, in their thirties, that they are unable to conceive now that they want to. About one couple in six experiences difficulty in achieving a successful pregnancy, making fertility a very widespread concern. Couples with fertility worries, although not physically unwell, are stressed by their situation. They tend to feel left behind by friends and relatives who have achieved a pregnancy easily. Their fertility situation becomes more and more central to their lives the longer it goes on. Decisions relating to housing and careers may have to be put on hold, and the couple consequently feel as though they are in limbo. Some couples find it helpful to be open about their fertility difficulties; they may share their experiences and feelings with others in the same situation through official or unofficial support groups or websites. For them, secrecy would be an additional stress. Other couples prefer to keep their situation as private as possible, feeling that, were others to become aware of their difficulties, their stress would be magnified. Privacy is hard to guarantee in Ireland, no matter how discreet clinics try to be.

This book is a valuable new resource for Irish couples with fertility concerns, particularly those who wish to retain a degree of privacy. It provides emotional support as well as very practical advice about available medical resources and how to access them.

Some (brief) medical advice is in order in this foreword. Although it is considered normal for a couple to take up to one year to achieve a pregnancy, it is no harm to see your general practitioner much sooner then this. The results of a semen analysis or of an FSH-level test (a blood-hormone test carried out on the second, third or fourth day of menstruation) may indicate the necessity of seeing a specialist straightaway – or, in the great majority of cases, the result of this test may be reassuringly normal. Expect a transvaginal ultrasound scan at the first visit to a fertility clinic and a plan to carry out a test of the fallopian tubes (a laparoscopy or a hysterosalpingogram). Do not be surprised if, after all tests have been completed, no absolute explanation for your failure to conceive is found and no treatment is recommended for the time being. Remember that surgery is occasionally necessary – to address fibroids, ovarian cysts or adhesions. Be aware that there are three categories of fertility treatment – ovulation induction, intrauterine insemination and IVF/ICSI – and that the very approximate success rates per cycle for these treatments are 10, 15 and 30 percent, respectively. Do not be offended if you encounter ageist attitudes; after a certain age (generally about thirty-eight), the woman's age becomes the key factor determining the likelihood of conception occurring. Fertility doctors have to be acutely aware of this 'biological clock' in deciding when to intervene, and with what treatment. Give the fertility clinic you attend feedback (positive or negative) about how well you feel they have treated you. Remember that the majority of couples who see a fertility specialist will have a baby, with or without treatment.

Dr John Waterstone
Cork Fertility Centre
March 2008

1

Getting Ready

Introduction

Congratulations! You have taken the first and most important step towards becoming a parent: you have made the decision to start trying to conceive.

Whether you need some time to come off contraception or are ready to go, it is strongly advisable for you to do some basic preparation before you start trying to conceive (TTC). Pregnancy is a wonderful time for most couples and it really doesn't last that long, so why not make the most of it by preparing your body, and your lives, as best you can? Some preparations, such as taking folic acid, will help ensure a healthy baby; others will help your body cope as best it can with the stresses and strains of pregnancy. You can't prepare for everything, and morning sickness and pelvic pain are inevitable for some, but starting with a healthy body will certainly help reduce the overall wear and tear that pregnancy can cause. Also, taking time to get to know your body and your menstrual cycle will help you take advantage of your fertile time and, hopefully, help you achieve a pregnancy sooner rather than later.

It's not just the women who need to prepare. Granted, a man's biological job is done before the baby is even created, but there are still steps that should be taken in advance to make sure you have the best quality and quantity of sperm available. And, men: TTC and pregnancy can be hard work at times, so you will need to be on hand for extra cooking, cleaning and hugging duties.

My own research has shown that over 80 percent of women (and I suspect an even greater proportion of men) do not follow pre-pregnancy dietary and exercise regimes as recommended by many books and websites. While it is important and beneficial to be in good health before you put your body

11

through the trials and tribulations of pregnancy, it is not necessarily a prerequisite to pregnancy if you are both fertile. In other words, being unfit and unhealthy may not stop you conceiving if you are fertile (although it is certainly a factor in some cases), but you might be taking risks with your baby's health and your own health if you do not follow certain basic steps before TTC.

For those with known conditions, such as endometriosis or PCOS, TTC may be a slightly more daunting prospect, and you may wish to talk to your doctor about steps you can take to improve your chances of conception. For those who wish to reverse a tubal ligation or vasectomy, the preparatory work will start long before the fun begins.

Whatever your situation, and however you want to approach the baby-making process, it is important to be armed with as much information as possible, to help both of you and your baby to make the best start together. And then the rest is up to you. Good luck!

Preparing your body

You should both start thinking about preparing your body for pregnancy about three months in advance. Men need to ensure that their sperm is of sufficient quality for conception, and women need to prepare their bodies for the nine months that lie ahead. Some steps, such as taking folic acid for the three months before and after conception, or having a rubella check, are strongly advised for all women, whereas many other steps are desirable but not as essential to the health of your baby.

It is a good idea for women to visit their GPs at least three months before they plan to start TTC. Your GP can carry out a rubella check and a smear test, and can test for any sexually transmitted infections (STIs) you may be concerned about. He or she can also check your iron levels and blood type. If you are on any medication, or have concerns about your weight, it is important to get advice from your GP at this stage, as both these things can have an effect on your fertility. If your partner is on medication or has any concerns about STIs, his weight or any other issues, it is a good idea for him to come with you.

Below is a list of things you may want to ask your GP about at your pre-pregnancy visit. Make sure to have a rubella check and a smear test if you are due one. If you have concerns about your weight, then you should also make sure to talk to your GP about your body mass index (BMI) and ask advice about how you can make changes to improve it. The other tests may not be essential for you, but if you have concerns about any of them, it is important to raise these with your GP at this visit.

Rubella check

This is probably the most important pre-pregnancy check of all. The rubella virus, while it does not cause serious illness in adults, can be very dangerous to an unborn child, especially during the first twelve weeks of pregnancy. Most Irish women have been vaccinated against rubella or have contracted the virus when they were younger, and so are probably immune. However, this immunity can wear off, so it is advisable to get tested for antibodies. If you do need to be vaccinated, you should wait at least three months before starting TTC.

Smear test

If you have not had a smear test in the last couple of years, or if you have had abnormalities in the past, you should think about getting one before you start TTC. While a smear test during pregnancy is usually considered safe, the results can sometimes be inconclusive, and if treatment is needed, it will not be started until at least six weeks post-partum. Bear in mind that smear-test results through your GP in Ireland can take up to six months to come back, so if you are planning to start TTC sooner than that, you may want to ask your GP or gynaecologist to have the sample tested privately so that you can get the results back within a few weeks.

BMI

If you are overweight or underweight, or more importantly if your body mass index (BMI) is outside the 'normal' range, you may be at risk of having fertility problems. Your BMI is a measure of the relationship between your weight and height and is calculated by dividing your weight in kilograms by your height in metres squared, e.g. 72kg/(1.72m x 1.72m) = 24.3. The VHI website has a free BMI calculator (which takes an input of feet, inches and pounds for those of you who are still 'unmetricated'): *www2.vhihealthe.com /topic/bmicalc*

BMI	ANALYSIS
18.4 and under	Underweight
18.5 to 24.9	Normal
25.0 to 29.9	Overweight
30 and over	Obese
40 and over	Morbidly obese

The table on page 13 gives a simple indication of a person's BMI and relative health. BMI is considered to give a good estimate of a person's weight adjusted for their height, and it tends to correlate with the percentage of fat on that person's body. However, as it does not take into account the distinction between muscle mass and fat, BMI is not a definitive guide to health status.

Fertility rates have been found to be lower, and miscarriage rates higher, in women who are overweight, and women with high BMIs have lower pregnancy rates, even with IVF. The reasons for the relationship between high BMIs and lower fertility aren't clearly defined, but most evidence points to the fact that a woman's hormonal balance can become disrupted when she is overweight. This can result in anovulation (no ovulation) or a poor quality of ovulation, where an insufficient amount of the hormones that support pregnancy are produced. Similarly, hormonal disruption can occur in women who are underweight (see Chapter 2 for more information on the hormones involved in the menstrual cycle and pregnancy).

Being under- or overweight will not necessarily prevent you from becoming pregnant, and if you are ovulating normally, then you should not worry. However, if your BMI is outside the normal range, then you may want to talk to your GP about how you can improve your BMI and your health before becoming pregnant. If you are not ovulating, then your GP may prescribe one of a number of fertility drugs to help you ovulate. He or she may advise you to lose or gain weight first if they feel it is necessary, and they may also prefer you to see a gynaecologist or fertility specialist so that you can be monitored while you are taking the fertility drugs. This is something that I recommend also. There is more information on ovulation problems, and medication that can help, in Chapter 6.

Studies have also shown that men who are overweight can suffer from poor sperm quality, and the higher the BMI, the more likely this is to happen. Excess weight in men has been linked with hormonal changes. If you are concerned that your weight may have an effect on your fertility, then talk to your GP about nutrional and other changes that you can make before you begin TTC.

Sexually transmitted infections (STIs)

During pregnancy, you will be routinely tested for any STI that could cause harm to your baby. Gonorrhoea, syphilis, hepatitis, herpes and HIV can all transfer to the baby in the birth canal during delivery, and syphilis, HIV and, in some cases, herpes can cross the placenta during pregnancy. If you or your partner are concerned about any of these infections, then you should mention it to your GP at your pre-pregnancy visit.

You may also want to get checked out for another STI, chlamydia, which can cause infertility. Chlamydia is the most common bacterial STI in the developed world. Three out of four of those who have it experience no symptoms, and if left untreated it can cause pelvic inflammatory disease, which can damage the fallopian tubes, the uterus and the surrounding tissue. In Ireland, there has been a three-fold increase in the number of known new cases of chlamydia per year since 1993. Chlamydia can be tested for by using a urine sample or a vaginal swab and, once diagnosed, can usually be treated successfully with antibiotics.

Blood group

It is a good idea to know the blood groups of both partners so that the Rhesus factor is known. A negative Rhesus factor in the female partner combined with a positive one in the male partner requires careful attention. This is because a woman who is Rhesus-negative may develop antibodies to her baby's blood if the baby is Rhesus-positive. Untreated, these antibodies can attack the blood cells of the foetus. This can result in the baby becoming anaemic or developing jaundice, or even more serious complications. This is easily prevented with an injection of a substance called RhoGAM, which blocks the formation of these antibodies in the mother.

Iron levels

During pregnancy, your body needs about two and a half times its usual amount of iron for you, your baby and the placenta. Low iron levels are a fairly common problem in pregnancy, even for women who do not usually suffer from anaemia. If you suspect that you may have low iron levels prior to becoming pregnant, you should start on an iron-rich diet, with iron supplements if necessary, so that you can prepare your body as well as possible for pregnancy. Your GP can test your iron levels using a simple blood test.

Toxoplasmosis

Toxoplasmosis is an infection caused by a parasite called toxoplasma gondii. The infection can be caught by eating anything that contains the parasite. This includes raw meat, unwashed fruit and vegetables, unpasteurised goat's milk and goat's-milk products, and anything that may have come into contact with cat faeces. Those infected with toxoplasmosis do not usually experience any symptoms (some mild flu-like symptoms may be present), and the infection rarely causes problems in healthy adults. However, it can cause eye and ear problems, brain damage, and even death to an unborn baby.

If you have a cat, don't panic. Most cat owners will have already come into contact with toxoplasmosis and will have developed an immunity to it. It is a good idea to ask your GP for a blood test, which will tell you if you have antibodies. If not, then there are several precautions you can take to keep both mother and baby safe.

§ Let someone else change the litter tray while you are TTC and until your baby is born. If this is not possible, make sure that you wear gloves when you are doing it.

§ Make sure that the tray is cleaned or scooped every day: the parasite doesn't become infectious until at least twenty-four hours after it lands in the tray.

§ Wear gloves when you are gardening.

§ Never give your cat or yourself raw or undercooked meat.

§ Wash all utensils and surfaces after preparing raw meat.

§ Avoid cured meats.

§ Avoid unpasteurised dairy products.

§ Wash all fruit and vegetables before use.

§ Avoid contact with stray or farm animals.

Listeria

Listeria is a species of bacteria found in soil, sewage and many raw and unprocessed foods. When eaten, it can cause listeriosis, which is a rare but potentially dangerous condition, especially to an unborn child. Listeriosis can cause miscarriage during the first trimester, growth restriction during the second trimester, and premature birth, meningitis and even death in the third trimester. The symptoms in non-pregnant women and men are fever, muscle aches, and gastrointestinal symptoms such as nausea or diarrhoea. If infection spreads to the nervous system, symptoms such as headache, stiff neck, loss of balance, confusion, decreased consciousness or convulsions can occur. Infected pregnant women usually only experience a mild, flu-like illness but are more susceptible to the disease due to hormonal changes that affect the immune system. If you are concerned, you can ask your GP for a simple blood test that can detect listeriosis, and this can then be treated with antibiotics, even if you have started TTC or are already pregnant.

For most women, taking some simple precautions both before and during pregnancy is enough to protect them against listeriosis:

§ Avoid soft cheeses (such as feta, Brie and Camembert) and blue-veined cheeses, as these are made with unpasteurised milk.

§ Avoid smoked meats and fish.

§ Avoid refrigerated patés and meat spreads; those that are canned or bought off the shelf are OK.

§ Avoid all shellfish and raw fish.

§ Wash all utensils and surfaces after preparing raw meat or fish.

§ Wash all fruit and vegetables before use.

Medication

Check with your GP that any medication you are on or are planning to take will not adversely affect your fertility and is considered safe during pregnancy. If you are planning a honeymoon or other holiday to an area for which you will need to take medical precautions, keep in mind that you may be advised not to TTC for a certain amount of time after you have stopped taking that medication.

Dental check

It is a good idea for women to have a dental check before starting TTC. Once you are pregnant, you won't be able to have X-rays, so any potential cavities will have to be left untreated until you have had your baby.

Nutrition

A sensible, balanced pre-pregnancy diet will give your body and your baby the best start in pregnancy. Pregnancy can be hard on your body (and on your stomach in particular), so the more you prepare before you conceive, the less of a toll pregnancy will take on you.

A healthy pre-pregnancy diet is of the utmost importance for women who suffer from morning sickness. The first trimester of pregnancy can take a serious toll on a woman's body, especially if she is one of those unlucky women who vomits constantly for the first two to three months of pregnancy. If you have never been pregnant before, then of course you don't know whether this will affect you, but it is better to be safe than sorry. And even if you have had a problem-free pregnancy in the past, you may not be so lucky in the future. I was lucky enough to suffer a 'normal' amount until my eighth pregnancy, and then I was hit with the full force of symptoms and threw up for two months!

During this time, it is pointless to tell women to eat a diet high in fibre, grains and fish when all they can stomach is white toast and mashed potato. So the more reserves your body has to draw on from before pregnancy, the better you will feel overall.

Diet

First and foremost, you need to make sure that you eat regular meals, with plenty of variety. Vitamins and mineral supplements are important, but the more you can get from your regular diet, the better.

Iron

Research suggests that 75 percent of women do not eat enough iron. As you will need increased amounts of iron in your diet during pregnancy, it is a good idea to start changing your diet in the months before you start TTC. Lean red meat is the best dietary source of iron. Other sources include fortified breakfast cereals, beans, eggs, apricots, prunes, figs, spinach and broccoli.

Vitamin C

In order to absorb iron into your blood, you need a good supply of vitamin C in your diet. Good sources of vitamin C include citrus fruits, kiwis, blackcurrants, mangoes and nectarines, and any drinks made from these fruits. Potatoes are also a fairly good source.

Calcium

You will need an extra store of calcium for your baby's teeth and bone development. The baby takes this from your body, so if you do not have enough calcium in your diet, your own stores will become depleted. Milk, yogurt and Cheddar cheese are the best sources of calcium. However, some medical practitioners consider that dairy products can have an adverse effect on fertility, so while you are TTC, it is best to get your calcium from green leafy vegetables, beans and fortified juices.

Omega-3 oils

Omega-3, a key fatty acid, has been found to aid fertility by reducing clotting and encouraging blood flow to the tissues, including the uterus. Omega-3 fatty acids also boost the immune system and have been found to reduce certain immune cells (NK, or natural killer, cells) which can prevent the embryo's implantation in the uterus. The omega-3 fatty acids, EPA and DHA, are also essential in foetal brain development. Omega-3 oils can be found in mackerel, herring, salmon, sardines and kippers or can be taken as a supplement.

Foods to avoid are those mentioned in the sections on toxoplasmosis and listeria. If you are a coffee or tea drinker, try to limit yourself to two cups a day. If you enjoy herbal teas, make sure that they are safe to drink when TTC and pregnant. If you are unsure about taking any herbs or supplements, then make sure to ask your GP if they are safe. Another product to avoid in large doses is soy, as it is thought to delay ovulation and cause longer menstrual cycles, and may also interfere with the sperm's journey to meet the egg.

Research has shown that a pre-pregnancy diet that is low in fibre and high in glycaemic load (those foods that have a significant effect on blood glucose levels) can increase the risk of gestational diabetes. This can affect the mother's health and can also result in a baby that is larger than normal, has low blood-sugar levels, or has jaundice at birth. Gestational diabetes is also related to women with high BMIs.

Vegetarians and vegans

Contrary to some popular beliefs, vegetarians and vegans can continue with their diets when TTC and pregnant. However, it is important to pay attention to what you eat to make sure that you are not lacking in any vital nutrients. Protein is an essential nutrient for the health of both mother and child. Vegetarians should make sure that their diets include plenty of dairy and soy products (just during pregnancy – go easy on both of these while TTC), lentils and beans. Vegans may need to work harder to ensure that their protein intake is adequate. Most individual plant-based protein sources lack all the essential amino acids, and so should be eaten in combination – pulses with grains or with seeds, for example. A dish made with lentils or chickpeas and served with brown rice is a good vegan protein source.

The other nutrient that vegetarians and vegans need to keep an eye on is vitamin B12, which is essential for the production of tissue and cells. It is also important for breastfeeding your baby. Vegetarians shouldn't have a problem getting enough B12 in their diets, as a single egg contains about 80 percent of your daily needs. However, there are few plant-based sources of B12, so if you are vegan, you may want to take a supplement. The recommended daily target is 1.5 micrograms per day.

Both vegetarians and vegans should try not to consume large amounts of soy when TTC. Some researchers believe that the phytoestrogens found in soy products can interfere with a woman's hormonal balance, leading to longer menstrual cycles and less-frequent ovulation. Regular amounts of soy are not thought to cause any problems: the 'large amounts' quoted are considered to be the equivalent of about three glasses of soy milk per day. Women are also advised to stay away from soy products around ovulation, as large amounts can hamper the sperm's journey to meet the egg.

Folic acid

It is essential that you start taking a folic-acid supplement three months before you plan to start TTC and continue to take this for the first three months of pregnancy. Folic acid is a B vitamin that helps prevent neural-tube defects (the neural tube is the part of a developing baby that becomes the brain and spinal cord). Studies suggest that up to 70 percent of neural-tube defects could be prevented if all women took a supplement of 400 micrograms of folic acid a day for the three months before and after conception. Folic acid can also be taken in the diet by eating fortified breakfast cereals, dried beans, leafy green vegetables and orange juice.

Prenatal vitamins

There is no harm in starting to take prenatal vitamins before you conceive. A good prenatal vitamin, such as Pregnacare, should contain at least 400 micrograms of folic acid, along with iron, zinc and B12 (B12 is especially important for vegetarians and vegans), and this will help you to build up your stores before you conceive.

Smoking, alcohol and drugs

Smoking, heavy drinking and recreational drugs are out. And that includes you too, men! Smoking, drinking and drugs, including some prescription drugs (ask your GP if you are on medication), can have an adverse effect on fertility for both partners. The exact effects of each of these on women's reproductive systems are not entirely clear but it is appears that all three can interfere with hormone production in women and that this can result in anovulation, poor quality of ovulation, and miscarriage. One study showed that female smokers take, on average, two months longer to conceive than non-smokers. However, once the woman has stopped smoking, her conception rate is similar to that of a woman who has never smoked. And of course, once you are pregnant you will need to stop smoking anyway.

The effect of all of the above, and in particular smoking, tends to be more detrimental to male fertility than female fertility. A US study has found that men who smoke can be 75 percent less likely to fertilise an egg in any given month compared to non-smokers. Smoking, heavy drinking and drugs have all been shown to contribute to a decline in sperm count, sperm motility and sperm morphology, all of which can cause male-factor infertility. The good news is that, because sperm take only about seventy-two days to be produced, any sperm made after you have stopped taking all of the above should be normal. So you need to stop about two and a half months before you plan to start TTC.

Many books and websites will tell you to stop drinking alcohol if you are TTC. While this may be an ideal, it is not always a realistic request, especially in Ireland. My advice to both of you is to have a few drinks once or twice a week if you want and not to worry about it. Set yourself a limit of, say, three drinks a night, and rest assured that by drinking in moderation you are unlikely to be doing much damage. (Although see the comments from Traditional Chinese Medicine practitioner Nina Liu on drinking when TTC, below.)

Traditional Chinese Medicine (TCM)

TCM, used either on its own or in conjunction with Western medicine, has been shown to improve fertility rates. Nina Liu, practitioner of Traditional Chinese Medicine at Melt in Temple Bar in Dublin, has helped many couples to conceive through the use of acupuncture, Chinese herbs and changes in diet. Nina explains that this works by rebalancing the body after it has been run down by poor diet, stress and medication, i.e. problems that most of us deal with in our everyday lives.

Infertility rates are lower in China than in the Western world, and Nina puts this down to the types of food that Chinese people eat. She recommends that a couple thinking about TTC should start making dietary changes about three months before they start TTC. Nina advises that couples cut down on alcohol, spicy foods, meat and dairy during this time, and make sure that their diets contains as many organic choices as possible. She also recommends that women avoid alcohol from day 10 to day 21 of their cycles when TTC, as this is the crucial stage for ovulation for most women.

Acupuncture can also aid fertility, even for couples with no known fertility problems. For those starting TTC for the first time, Nina recommends acupuncture for general health rebalancing, as most people suffer from some level of stress in their lives. A programme of acupuncture sessions for both partners once a week for the two- to three-month period before starting TTC will help maximise both your health and your fertility. While TTC, Nina recommends that the woman has acupuncture on days 1, 4, 13 and 21 of her cycle in order to ensure the best possible quality of ovulation and hormonal balance, in order to aid conception and protect against miscarriage.

Be realistic

Pregnancy does not always happen as soon as you want it to, so don't set yourself targets that you may not be able to maintain over several months. Don't deprive yourself of life's simple pleasures (unless those pleasures are smoking or taking recreational drugs!). After all, you still have to live your life while you are TTC.

Stopping contraception

The pill

The pill contains the hormones oestrogen and progestogen, which prevent ovulation. Once you stop taking the pill, the hormones should be out of your body within a few days. After that, your body will start to produce its own hormones and you will start ovulating again. For some women, this happens immediately; others can take several weeks or months to start menstruating normally again. It shouldn't matter whether you were on the pill for a few months or for ten years: as soon as you stop taking it, your body should start trying to get back to normal. However, if you had problems with your cycle before you started taking the pill, those problems may present themselves again. If you are concerned, you should talk to your GP.

The contraceptive injection

The contraceptive injection contains the hormone progestogen, which prevents ovulation for at least three months after the shot is administered. The average woman will ovulate about six to nine months after their last shot. The length of time you have been having the injections has no effect on how long it will take for ovulation to return. Some women have reported taking as long as eighteen months for their periods to return. If you have still not had a period nine months after your last shot, contact your GP or gynaecologist, who may be able to help regulate your hormone levels so that you can start ovulating again.

Intra-uterine device (IUD)

An IUD is a small, T-shaped contraceptive device that is surgically implanted into a woman's uterus. IUDs work by preventing the egg from being fertilised by the sperm. An IUD causes no hormonal changes to the body and, once it is removed, your menstrual cycle should continue as normal; pregnancy is possible after your next ovulation.

Intra-uterine system (IUS)

An IUS is similar to an IUD but has added protection in that it releases the hormone prostogen daily, which alters the endometrial lining so that implantation of a fertilised egg cannot take place. Once the IUS is removed, you should start menstruating normally again, but because of the hormonal changes, this may take several weeks.

The implant

The implant is a small rod that is inserted under the skin. It releases the hormone progestogen, which stops ovulation. Once the rod is removed, your fertility should return to normal, although, again because of the hormonal changes, this can take a few weeks.

The patch

The patch is similar to a small plaster and releases the hormones oestrogen and progestogen, which are absorbed through the skin to prevent ovulation. As with the pill, as soon as you stop using the patch, your body should start trying to get back to normal. It usually takes one to three months for periods to return to normal after the last patch.

Vaginal ring

The vaginal ring is a flexible ring that is inserted into the vagina for three weeks of every month. It releases the hormones oestrogen and progestogen, which prevent ovulation. Again, like the pill and the patch, once you stop using the vaginal ring, you should expect your periods to return to normal within about one to three months.

Diaphragm/condom

The diaphragm or cap is similar to a condom in that both are purely barrier methods of contraception, preventing sperm from reaching the egg. Once you stop using a diaphragm or a condom, you can conceive any time you have sex during your fertile time.

Tubal-ligation reversal

Tubal ligation, also known as 'having your tubes tied', is a permanent method of birth control. During a tubal ligation, a woman's fallopian tubes are cut or blocked by various methods so that the eggs cannot travel down the tubes to meet the sperm. If a woman subsequently decides that she wants to have a baby, she has two options: IVF, or a tubal-ligation reversal.

With IVF, the eggs are collected directly from the ovaries and fertilised in a lab by the sperm. The fertilised embryos are then transferred into the woman's uterus, thereby bypassing the need for the eggs or embryos to travel down the fallopian tube into the uterus.

A tubal reversal involves removing the damaged part of the tube and sewing the 'good' ends back together. There must be enough length in the tube to reattach it. This works best for women under forty, who have had their original surgery less than ten years previously, and for whom only small sections of the tube have been damaged by the previous surgery. The tubal reversal can be done under general anaesthetic with a single incision to the abdomen. A small lighted telescope, known as a laparoscope, is inserted into the incision, and the surgeon can then view the tubes on a monitor. The tools to repair the tubes can then be inserted into the incision, and a further incision may be made if necessary.

Pregnancy rates after tubal reversal depend on the method of tubal ligation that was performed in the first place, along with the age of the woman and the fertility of her partner. There is a greater risk of ectopic pregnancy after tubal reversal, where the embryo implants in the fallopian tube instead of in the uterus. There is more information on ectopic pregnancy in Chapter 9. If you are concerned about this, call your doctor immediately.

Vasectomy reversal

A vasectomy is a minor surgical procedure that involves cutting each of the two tubes, the vas deferens, which carry sperm from the testicles to the penis. After a vasectomy, there is no sperm present in the seminal fluid ejaculated during sex. If a man subsequently decides he wants to try for a baby, his two options are IVF and vasectomy reversal.

In order to obtain sperm for IVF, a testicular biopsy is performed, during which sperm is extracted directly from the testicle. A single sperm is then injected directly into an egg using a technique called intracytoplasmic sperm injection (ICSI – see Chapter 7). The fertilised egg is then transferred directly into the woman's uterus.

A vasectomy reversal involves rejoining each vas deferens. The standard

24

vasectomy reversal operation is called a vasovasostomy, and involves cutting the scrotum on each side so that the surgeon can remove any scar tissue from the vas deferens and then sew the two ends back together. A more complicated procedure, known as a vasoepididymostomy, involves joining the vas deferens directly to a tube called the epididymis. This technique can bypass any blockages in the vas deferens that may have arisen from a previous vasectomy or reversal operation.

The sooner a vasectomy reversal is done after the original vasectomy, the more successful it is likely to be. There is approximately an 80 percent success rate if the reversal is done within three years. This drops to 30 percent if fifteen years or more have passed since the vasectomy.

Factors affecting sperm quality

There are many factors that affect sperm quality. These include temperature, toxins, medication, diet, weight and genetic factors. All of these can decrease the number of sperm produced (sperm count), the ability of the sperm to move properly (sperm motility) and the shape of the sperm (sperm morphology), resulting in sub-fertility or infertility. Luckily, many of these factors are within your control, and the effects of them can be reversed.

Unlike women, who are born with all the eggs they will ever produce, men produce sperm approximately every seventy-two days. This means that, if a lifestyle or environmental factor is interfering with a man's sperm production, once this external factor has ceased, all sperm produced subsequently should not be affected. So, if your sperm count is below normal because you are a heavy smoker, then about seventy-two days after you have stopped smoking, you should see an improvement in your sperm count. Of course, things may not be that simple, as multiple factors may be involved. However, there are certain steps that you can take to improve your sperm quality and make sure you are maximising your chances of conception:

1. *Stop smoking*
   As mentioned previously, this can dramatically reduce your sperm quality.

2. *Avoid recreational drugs*
   Marijuana can decrease sperm count, sperm motility and sperm morphology. Cocaine and opiates can contribute to erectile dysfunction, and amphetamines can decrease sex drive.

3. *Limit alcohol intake*
   Try to limit your alcohol consumption to three drinks, twice a week.

4. *Avoid saunas, jacuzzis and hot baths*
   Avoid all sources of excessive or prolonged heat, as this can affect sperm production and damage sperm quality.

5. *Take stretch breaks*
   Prolonged sitting at work, at home or in your car can increase your scrotal temperature and impair sperm production.

6. *Watch out for toxins*
   Be careful when handling workplace and household chemicals, as these may reduce sperm count and motility. Wear gloves and protective clothing where possible.

7. *Check all medications with your doctor*
   Many prescription medications can temporarily reduce your fertility.

8. *Ensure a healthy BMI*
   Men who are overweight have been shown to have lower sperm quality than those who have BMIs within the normal limits.

9. *Include essential vitamins in your diet*
   Vitamins C and E are powerful antioxidants that protect the sperm and contribute to increased sperm concentration and better sperm motility. Vitamin C is found in citrus fruits, and vitamin E is found in walnuts, almonds and vegetable oils such as sunflower and safflower. Zinc is also an essential mineral for the healthy formation and maturation of sperm. It can be found in pumpkin seeds, shellfish and red meat.

So you can see by now that TTC really is a joint venture between the man and the woman. When you consider the fact that male-factor infertility accounts for a similar percentage of cases of fertility problems as female-factor infertility, you can see just how important it is for dad to be in as good shape as mum. So now you know what you need to do, off you go and get yourselves organised, and then the real fun can begin!

2

It's all about timing

Introduction

Many couples are surprised to learn that there is only a short window of opportunity for pregnancy each month. There are approximately three to five days each month when sex can result in pregnancy. This chapter will help you to become familiar with your menstrual cycle and your fertility signs so that you can maximise your chances of conceiving.

There is a widely held belief that ovulation occurs on day 14 of the menstrual cycle. This is the *average* day of ovulation for women with twenty-eight-day cycles, but there is really no such thing as a typical cycle. The length of a normal menstrual cycle varies from about twenty-two days to about thirty-six days, and this varies from woman to woman. Moreover, for each woman, it can also vary from cycle to cycle, depending on changes in lifestyle and hormone levels.

For example, imagine you have a twenty-six-day cycle. You may assume that you ovulate on day 14, and so you have sex on that day. However, if your actual ovulation day is day 12, then you will have already ovulated by the time you have sex and will have no chance of conceiving.

Learning to observe your fertility signs will help you take the guesswork out of TTC. If you can pinpoint your exact day of ovulation, there is no need to worry that you have missed the boat. It will also help you to become familiar with your cycle and with your body, so that if there is a problem, it can be more easily diagnosed and treated.

The menstrual cycle explained

If you want to determine your most fertile time, you need a general understanding of the changes that occur in your body during your menstrual cycle. This is also vital when trying to pinpoint hormonal or ovulatory problems: if you understand your body's signals, you will be able to help your medical practitioner help you. A good understanding of the menstrual cycle and the interplay of the hormones that drive it will also help you navigate the minefield of advice that is available on Internet message boards.

The menstrual cycle is usually divided into two distinct phases: the follicular or pre-ovulation phase and the luteal or post-ovulation phase. Each is approximately two weeks long, although this varies from woman to woman and can vary from cycle to cycle for each woman. The variation is particularly large in the follicular phase, which can be anything from eight days to about a month long, whereas the luteal phase can last from about eight to sixteen days.

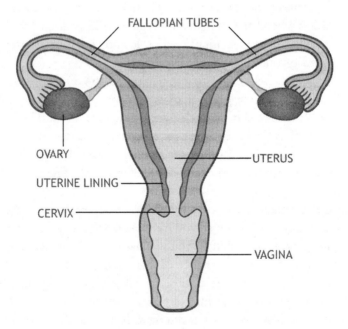

Fig. 2.1 The female reproductive system

Follicular phase

The first day of your period is the first day of your menstrual cycle. This is usually abbreviated to 'CD1' (cycle day 1) online. Some women may experience some spotting for a day (or in some cases for several days) before their period begins: this is not the first day of menstruation. CD1 is the first day of bright-red bleeding. The bleeding is caused by the shedding of your uterine lining (or endometrium), which has built up to full thickness in preparation for pregnancy during the previous cycle. If no pregnancy has occurred, then the endometrium sheds itself in the form of menstrual bleeding. At this stage of your cycle, none of the key hormones are present in any significant quantity.

Just before the cycle begins, the pituitary gland (located in the brain) starts to produce low levels of FSH (follicle-stimulating hormone). FSH is the hormone that stimulates the growth of ovarian follicles. Every woman is born with all the eggs she will ever use, and each egg is encased in its own follicle in the ovary. Each cycle, about ten to fifteen follicles begin to mature, and they compete against each other to become the dominant follicle. Ovulation occurs when the dominant follicle releases an egg.

When FSH begins to be released, the follicles start to mature. As they develop, the follicles secrete increasing amounts of oestrogen. This oestrogen initiates the production of a new endometrial layer. When one (or occasionally two) of the follicles begins to emerge as dominant, the others start to disintegrate. Once it is dominant, the follicle increases its oestrogen production dramatically, and this stimulates the cervix to produce fertile-quality cervical mucous (or CM). This CM is necessary for the survival and transport of sperm: sperm can survive and swim for up to five days in fertile CM; without it, they live for only a few hours. (There is more on recognising fertile CM later in the chapter.)

Once oestrogen levels reach a threshold, this stimulates the pituitary gland to release a surge of luteinising hormone (LH). This LH surge triggers ovulation, and the follicle will release the egg approximately twelve to thirty-six hours later. (There is more about pinpointing the time of this surge later in the chapter.) Once it has been released, the egg will survive for between six and twenty-four hours before it disintegrates, if it is not fertilised.

Luteal phase

Once the follicle releases the egg, it starts to form the corpus luteum (literally, 'yellow body') on the inside of the ovarian wall. The corpus luteum secretes large amounts of progesterone and lesser amounts of oestrogen. Progesterone plays a vital role in converting the endometrium into a form that will be receptive to the implantation of an embryo. At this time, fertile CM dries up, and the rise in progesterone curtails the production of LH and FSH. These hormones remain low until near the end of the cycle.

If no pregnancy has occurred, the corpus luteum starts to disintegrate towards the end of the luteal phase. If an embryo has implanted in the endometrium at this stage, it will produce the pregnancy hormone HCG (human chorionic gonadotropin), and the corpus luteum will remain viable for several more months. If the corpus luteum dies, the drop in progesterone and oestrogen production signals the endometrial lining to break down and the pituitary gland to start producing FSH, and the cycle starts all over again.

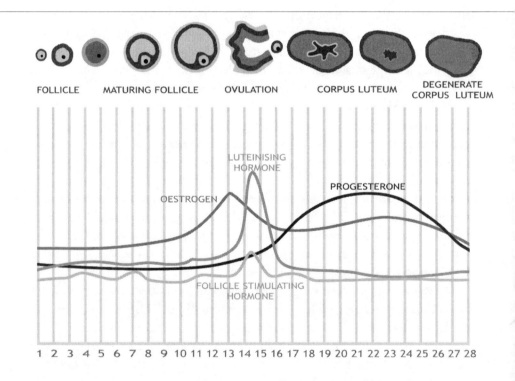

Fig. 2.2 The menstrual cycle

Menstrual-cycle summary

So, for those who have skipped the science bit, here is the menstrual cycle in brief:

§ On day 1 of your period (CD1), your uterine lining starts to shed and your body produces FSH.

§ This stimulates the development of the follicles in your ovaries which contain your eggs; about ten to fifteen of these begin to develop every cycle.

§ As these follicles mature, they release oestrogen, which helps build up your uterine lining and also stimulates the production of fertile cervical mucous that is necessary for the survival and transportation of sperm.

§ One of these follicles will eventually become dominant, and the others will disintegrate.

§ When oestrogen production reaches a certain level, the pituitary gland releases a surge of LH (luteinising hormone).

§ The LH surge instructs the follicle to release the egg, and about twelve to thirty-six hours later you will ovulate.

§ Once the follicle releases the egg, it becomes the corpus luteum.

§ This secretes large amounts of progesterone, which builds the uterine lining in preparation for implantation.

§ If no implantation occurs, the corpus luteum starts to disintegrate, the drop in progesterone triggers the uterine lining to disintegrate, and the cycle begins again.

Anovulatory and irregular cycles

There are certain times during a woman's menstrual life when she may not ovulate: during adolescence, pregnancy, breastfeeding and perimenopause. These phases of anovulation are completely normal. However, outside of these scenarios, if a woman has got her period, she may well assume that she is ovulating, whereas this is not necessarily the case. In fact, it is not unusual for a woman to have the odd anovulatory cycle. There are certain situations which can affect the body to such an extent that it does not produce enough oestrogen to trigger the process of ovulation. Illness, travel, strenuous exer-

31

cise, weight gain or loss, stress and certain medical conditions can affect the balance of the menstrual cycle.

All of the above factors can also delay ovulation, resulting in an irregular cycle. However, the most common cause of ongoing irregular cycles is an underlying hormonal balance, which can usually be treated. There is more on this in Chapter 6.

Fertility signs

It is often thought that the day of ovulation is the best day to have sex that will result in pregnancy. This is not strictly true, as the egg survives for only six to twenty-four hours after ovulation before disintegrating. The optimal situation is when the sperm are waiting in the fallopian tube, ready to fertilise the egg as soon as it is released. In order for this to happen, you need at least a couple of days' warning that ovulation is imminent. This is possible when you learn to observe your fertile signs.

There are four main indicators that you are in your fertile period, that is the period leading up to and including ovulation. The signs to look out for are: changes in cervical mucous, changes in cervical position, an LH surge, and changes in waking temperature.

Changes in cervical mucous (CM)

If you've never observed your cervical fluid before, then you may not be aware of its cyclical nature, even if you have noticed changes in volume and texture over a period of time. Throughout your menstrual cycle, your CM changes in response to the hormonal changes in your body. We have already seen that a sharp increase in oestrogen levels triggers the production of fertile-quality CM. Similarly, the other hormonal changes affect the consistency and amount of CM that your body produces. It is important to note that all CM prior to ovulation can be considered fertile to some extent, but that it is the slippery, stretchy type that signals that ovulation is on its way and that is also most conducive to the survival and transportation of sperm.

The way in which you observe your CM is up to you. The most accurate method is to insert your finger into your vagina and collect some CM. However, some women find this too uncomfortable, too messy, or simply too much hassle. For the purposes of observing changes in CM, it is absolutely fine to collect it on some toilet paper and have a look at it that way. Make sure you wipe before and after going to the toilet, as you will get a better idea of what's there.

As your menstruation comes to an end, you will probably have a period of dryness or possibly just a small amount of moisture at the vaginal opening. After a few days, you may notice a slight increase in CM, and that it has a sticky or paste-like consistency. The next type of CM you will have should feel wet and have a creamy texture, like hand lotion. As you approach ovulation and your oestrogen levels peak, you should notice CM that looks like egg white (this is usually abbreviated on Internet message boards to 'EWCM'). It is slippery and stretches to more than a quarter of an inch when held between the thumb and forefinger, or between two sheets of toilet paper. This is your most fertile CM – whenever you see this, it is time to get down to business. Most women will have between two and four days of EWCM. As soon as you have ovulated, your CM tends to dry up, and it may remain dry or slightly moist until the end of your cycle. You may also notice that it gets sticky a day or two before your period is due.

STAGE OF CYCLE	CERVICAL MUCOUS
Menstruation	Bleeding
Post-menstruation	Dry or slightly moist
Pre-fertile period	Sticky or paste-like
	Creamy or lotiony
Fertile period	Slippery, stretchy, like egg white
Post-ovulation	Dry or sticky

Anecdotal evidence suggests that creamy or lotiony CM during the two-week wait (the time between ovulation and when you can test for pregnancy) may indicate pregnancy. In my experience, there does tend to be more CM than usual during the luteal phase of a pregnant cycle. However, I have also noticed this during some non-pregnant cycles, so it is not a sure-fire sign of pregnancy by any means. If only there was such a thing . . .

Changes in cervical position (CP)

The cervix is that lower, narrow portion of the uterus that joins the vagina. As with CM, the CP undergoes changes at specific times during the menstrual cycle, and observation and tracking of these changes can be used to predict ovulation.

I have to say that monitoring of this fertility sign is not for the faint-hearted, and it is something I tried only a couple of times. It is not essential to track your CP, but if your other fertility signs are not conclusive – if you are not producing much CM, not having much of an LH surge, or your waking temperatures are not providing an accurate pattern of ovulation – then it is well worth keeping an eye on your CP.

As with taking your temperature and testing for an LH surge, you should check your cervix at the same time every day. Make sure that you wash your hands first. Insert one or two fingers into your vagina, and push upwards and backwards until you reach the top: this is your cervix. If your cervix is relatively easy to reach, then the position is low; if it is harder to reach, then the position is high. You also need to check whether your cervix feels soft or firm, open or closed, and wet or not. These are all relative characteristics that you will only begin to identify when you have checked your cervix on a regular basis over a number of cycles.

Prior to ovulation, your cervix will feel relatively firm (like touching the tip of your nose), dry to the touch, low and closed. As you approach ovulation, your cervix will become increasingly soft and moist, and the entrance will start to open and rise in response to the high levels of oestrogen in your body. Around this time, the cervix will release fertile-quality CM. Once you have ovulated, your cervix will return to the low, hard, closed and dry position.

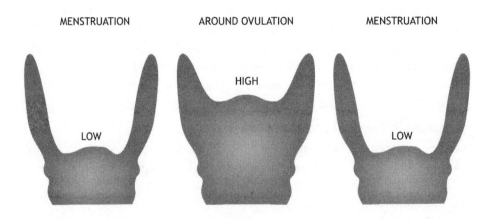

MENSTRUATION AROUND OVULATION MENSTRUATION

HIGH

LOW   LOW

Fig. 2.3 Cervical positions

LH surge

As we have seen, approximately twelve to thirty-six hours before you ovulate, your body will experience a surge of LH. Changes in the level of LH in your system can be detected in urine, and you can test for this using ovulation-prediction kits (OPKs). (These are made up of individual tests, and are usually sold in packs, hence the name 'kit'.) OPKs are used in exactly the same way as home-pregnancy tests (HPTs) – either you pee directly on to the stick, or you can collect your urine in a cup and then dip the stick, or the strip, into it.

The main difference between HPTs and OPKs lies in how you read them. With HPTs, a second line, however faint, is a positive result. In order to get a positive result on an OPK, the test line has to be *as dark as* the control line. In fact, your LH levels may be high enough throughout your cycle to show a second line on an OPK at any time. It is only when this line becomes as dark as the control line that you have had your LH surge.

Unlike with HPTs, it is better to use OPKs in the afternoon or evening. This is because your LH surge usually begins in the morning, so it is more likely that you will catch it if you test later in the day. I usually test when I come in from work at about 6 PM.

It can be difficult to read the results on an OPK. Sometimes the test line looks almost as dark as the control line, and if it is considerably darker than the previous day, then there is a tendency to assume that it is positive. Most likely what has happened in this case is that you have caught the beginning or the end of the surge, and if you test again in a couple of hours (or had tested a couple of hours previously), the test would be positive. It may take you a couple of cycles to be able to read your OPKs with confidence.

When you should start testing for your LH surge depends on the usual length of your cycles. If you have been monitoring your cycles for a while, then you may have some idea when you ovulate. If you have no idea, then it is best to take the shortest cycle you have had in the last six months and use that as the basis for when you will start testing, to make sure you don't miss the surge on another short cycle. The chart below will give you an idea of what day of your cycle you should start testing.

Cycle length	21	22	23	24	25	26	27	28	29	30
Start testing	5	5	6	7	8	9	10	11	12	13
Cycle length	31	32	33	34	35	36	37	38	39	40
Start testing	14	15	16	17	18	19	20	21	22	23

If your OPK is positive most or all of the time, then it is possible that you have polycystic ovary syndrome (PCOS). PCOS is an endocrine disorder which results in constantly high levels of LH in the system. There is more about PCOS and the available treatments for it in Chapter 6.

Checking for an LH surge with OPKs is probably the simplest method of predicting ovulation, and it is the one that most newcomers seem to prefer. However, it is possible (although rare) to have an LH surge and still not ovulate, so if you have any doubts, you should cross-check your OPK results with your other fertility signs and use a temperature chart to make sure that ovulation has taken place.

Other methods of ovulation prediction

As well as OPKs, there are other devices available that can tell you that your body is gearing up to ovulate. They are usually referred to as fertility monitors, but different types use different methods of detecting impending ovulation. They range in price from about €20 to several hundred euro, so they tend to be bought as an investment by those who have tried other methods unsuccessfully or those who are planning more than one baby. It is important to remember that, while these monitors can tell you when you are about to ovulate, the readings do not guarantee that you will actually ovulate. If you are concerned that you may not be ovulating, then you should chart your temperatures as well.

Urine monitor

Urine monitors, usually called fertility monitors, are hand-held electronic devices that measure the levels of oestrogen and LH in your system, and give you a reading of 'low', 'high' or 'peak' fertility. These monitors require a monthly purchase of test sticks or discs, so they can be a costly investment. At a specified time each day, you collect your urine in a cup and dip the stick in the cup, or drop your urine onto a test disc. The monitor will then return a reading based on your hormone levels. Urine fertility monitors are available from *www.smartpaddy.ie* and cost about €140. The test sticks cost about €30 for twenty sticks.

Electrolyte monitor

These monitors measure the electrolytes in saliva or cervical mucous, or both, by means of a probe attached to an electronic device, and can predict ovulation from five to seven days in advance. Some monitors will store your readings in their memory so you don't have to make a note of them every day – and some even have the facility to upload the readings to your computer. These cost several hundred euro but do not need any additional purchase apart from a battery. I can't recommend any sites that sell them, although I have seen them on eBay.

Salivary ferning test

Saliva monitors, also known as saliva microscopes or ovulation monitors, show a 'ferning' pattern when you are approaching ovulation. First thing every morning, you take a bit of saliva on the tip of your finger and smear it on to the lens of the microscope. After about five minutes, you can look at the monitor and determine whether or not you see a ferning pattern. These monitors are available from *www.saveontests.com* for US$25.

Changes in waking temperature

When you ovulate, your temperature rises. This is due to the large amounts of progesterone that the corpus luteum produces. A woman's preovulatory waking temperature ranges from approximately 36 to 36.5 degrees Celsius, and this rises to about 36.5 to 37 degrees within a day or so after ovulation. These temperatures stay high until the corpus luteum starts to break down and stops producing progesterone. This is usually the day before you will get your period, although it can happen on the same day, or a couple of days later. If you are pregnant, then your temperatures will remain elevated through the time of your expected period and beyond, as the HCG produced by your body will signal the corpus luteum to keep producing progesterone.

It is essential to take your waking temperature at the same time every morning, as your temperature will be different at different times of the morning. You will also need a basal body thermometer or one that is calibrated to two decimal places, as even small changes in temperature can be significant.

When reading temperature charts, it is important to look at the pattern of temperatures, as opposed to the individual highs and lows. One temperature in isolation will not tell you anything, as many factors, such as alcohol consumption and illness, can affect your waking temperature. So don't worry if one temperature is higher or lower than you expected: the chart will probably even out over the next few days.

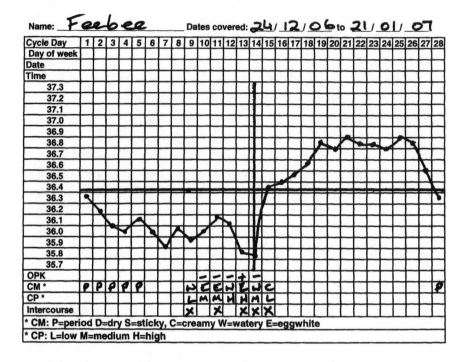

Fig. 2.4 A typical temperature chart

Charting your waking (or basal body) temperatures will give you a very accurate picture of when you ovulate. However, this needs to be done over a number of cycles, as one cycle in isolation will only tell you when you have already ovulated. If you look at your temperature charts over a period of time, then you will be able to pinpoint your usual day of ovulation (to within a couple of days) and use that information to predict ovulation in your next cycle.

On an individual cycle basis, your temperature chart is a useful tool for corroborating your other fertility signs, and is the only sure-fire way of knowing that you have actually ovulated. All the other signs indicate that you are about to ovulate but cannot guarantee that this will actually happen. Once you see a sustained temperature rise (over three days or more), you can be sure that the follicle has released an egg, has become the corpus luteum, and has started producing progesterone.

If your cycles are irregular, then your temperature charts may not be useful for predicting ovulation. However, they will tell you when you have ovulated, so you will know what phase of your cycle you are in. If you know you have made it into the luteal phase, then at least you can relax a bit (or as much as is possible during the two-week wait!). There is more about charting your cycles in Chapter 3.

Another, less reliable, indication is a pain in either or both sides of your lower abdomen around the expected time of ovulation. This pain is called Mittelschmerz (German for 'middle pain') and can last anything from a few minutes to several hours. There are several possible causes for this – swelling of the follicles, the egg bursting out of the ovary, the release of blood or fluid from the ruptured follicle – and it cannot be used to determine the time of ovulation, as it can occur before, during or after ovulation. It is, however, a useful secondary fertility sign that can be used to cross-check the primary fertility indicators.

What if your fertility signs disagree?

If you are keeping track of more than one fertility sign, then it is important to remember that none of them can pinpoint the exact time of ovulation, and that they are accurate to within three days. So you may have a positive OPK and your temperature may not rise for another three days. This means that you could have ovulated the day after the positive OPK or the day after that. Some people will ovulate the same day as the positive OPK, some two days later. Some people will have fertile cervical mucous the day of, and the day after, ovulation, some only up until a day or two before. Similarly, CP and waking temperature will vary amongst women.

If your fertility signs vary to the extent that you cannot match them at all, then the most reliable one to use is your temperature chart. Your temperature will only show a sustained shift once you have ovulated. If you are concerned that your CP, your CM or your LH surge are completely at odds with your temperature chart, then you should see your medical practitioner, who can test your hormone levels on day 3 of your cycle, and again at seven days past ovulation (7 DPO), to see if there are any imbalances that may be affecting your cycle. There is more on this in Chapter 5.

Timed intercourse

In theory, having sex at any time during your fertile period can result in pregnancy. This is because sperm can survive for up to five days in fertile CM. Of course, this is only in an optimal environment, and as we have no way of measuring that, it is best to have a plan.

No matter how much you are looking forward to endless, contraception-free sex, I can guarantee you that a few months into your every-night-for-two-weeks routine, you will be ready to throw a heavy object at the next person who tells you: 'At least you'll have fun trying!' So how often should you have sex, and when should you start?

A general rule of thumb is that you should have sex on every day that you see EWCM. However, as this may be hard for some women to identify, especially at first, and because sometimes life tends to get in the way, it is better to have a more definite plan.

If you are dealing with a normal sperm count (or if you are assuming a normal sperm count), then it is OK to have sex every day. If a sperm analysis has shown a low count, then it is better to try every second day, in order to give the count a chance to build up as much as possible. If your own sperm analysis has shown another sub-fertile result, then you should talk to your medical practitioner about how best to optimise your chances of conceiving.

The man should try to abstain from any sort of ejaculation for three days before your first attempt. You should start trying four or five days before you expect to ovulate. If you have no idea when you ovulate, then you should take the shortest cycle you have had in the last six months and use the chart below to calculate your start day.

Cycle length	21	22	23	24	25	26	27	28	29	30
Start trying	5	5	6	7	8	9	10	11	12	13
Cycle length	31	32	33	34	35	36	37	38	39	40
Start trying	14	15	16	17	18	19	20	21	22	23

You can try every day, or every second day, until you see EWCM, notice a change in your CP, or get a positive OPK. Then it is best to try every day up to and including the last day of EWCM, the day your cervix has returned to the low, hard, closed and dry position, two days after your positive OPK, or the day you notice a temperature shift. Although the temperature shift happens *after* you have ovulated, there is a chance that the egg may still be alive the next day. As it survives for about twelve hours after ovulation, if you have ovulated during the night or if more than one egg has been released, you may still be in with a chance. It is not necessary to try the day of the temperature rise, but it does cover all bases.

Tips and theories

There is a lot of talk online about the best way to get those sperm swimming up to meet the egg, and plenty of tips available on how to give them a helping hand. The general consensus is that the missionary position is best to ensure that the majority of sperm are released into the cervix and don't have to battle gravity as their journey begins. However, the truth is that as long as there is fertile CM present, the sperm should be able to reach their destination regardless of sexual position. You may also read that putting a pillow under your bum or hoisting your legs in the air for half an hour after sex will help the sperm travel towards your cervix. Although neither of these things will do you any harm, and may indeed move the sperm in the right direction, an adequate amount of EWCM is all they need to help them along their way: without it, the sperm may never reach their destination, no matter how much you help them reach your cervix.

A popular, ready-made plan for those who have been pregnant before is the 'Sperm Meets Egg Plan'. All the details are here: *www.pregnancyloss.info /sperm_meets_egg_plan.htm*.

Trying for a girl or a boy

The Shettles method of sex selection is based on the theory that 'male' sperm swim faster but have shorter lives than 'female' sperm. Therefore, in order to conceive a boy, a couple would have sex on the day of ovulation: because the male sperm swim faster, they would reach the egg first. To conceive a girl, the couple would have sex up until a few days before ovulation: by the time of ovulation, the male sperm would have died, but the longer-living females would still be there to fertilise the egg. The Shettles method also suggests that male sperm favour an alkaline environment, whereas female sperm thrive in an acidic environment. Therefore, by making the vagina more alkaline (via female orgasm, or douching with baking soda prior to intercourse), male sperm will survive over female sperm. In order to ensure an acidic vagina, women should avoid orgasm and douche with white vinegar before ovulation.

Although proponents of the Shettles method profess a 75 percent success rate, anecdotal evidence suggests that it is closer to 50 percent. One thing is for sure: douching and abstaining from intercourse at your most fertile time will definitely decrease your chances of conception.

The two-week wait

So you've watched for all your fertility signs, you've got down to business at all the right times, and you've ovulated. Congratulations, you are now on the two-week wait (2ww)! You have only about twelve sleeps to go before you can test to see if all your hard work has paid off. Sounds simple enough, eh? Well, if you find waiting out the next twelve to fourteen days easy, please drop me a line and tell me how you've done it.

The 2ww can seem like an unending cycle of conflicting signs and symptoms, of emotional highs and lows, where the mind can focus on nothing but the predetermined (yet unknown) outcome. In my experience, it is no use telling women to stop obsessing: it is impossible for them to do so. If the 2ww is new to you, you will be overcome with excitement and daydreams for the months ahead; if you have been suffering the 2ww for some time, then the desperation you feel may supersede everything else in your life.

Pregnancy symptoms that women have reported during a successful 2ww include sore boobs, heartburn, burping, tiredness, metallic taste in mouth, creamy CM, cramps and weepiness. It is, of course, possible to have all of these symptoms every month and still not be pregnant. If you have never kept an eye out for them, you will be unaware whether they are indeed pregnancy symptoms or are in fact completely unrelated. It is not uncommon for women to spend several hours a day poking and prodding their breasts, watching every bodily function for a twinge or an ache, and Googling said twinges and aches for any pregnancy-related evidence. I have to confess to spending many, many months Googling '3 DPO symptoms' (three days past ovulation) and other pointless terms – until I started getting my own blog posts as search results!

The first thing you have to accept about the 2ww is that you will get no pregnancy symptoms until an embryo has implanted itself in the uterine lining. This is because pregnancy symptoms are caused by an increase in the level of the hormone HCG, and this only occurs when an embryo starts to implant. Implantation happens from approximately 6 to 10 DPO. So until then, all the 'symptoms' you are having are unrelated to pregnancy – or are perhaps just a sign that you have ovulated.

Once you do reach the halfway stage of the 2ww, you are free to obsess! However, it is unlikely that you will get any strong symptoms until a week or two after you have had a positive test. As a veteran of eight pregnancies, I can confirm that none of my 2wws have yielded conclusive symptoms. Unusual tiredness is the one I would put most trust in, followed by heartburn and burping. Unfortunately, all of the other 'symptoms' are also signs of impending menstruation. Yes, the greatest con of TTC is that pregnancy symptoms are almost identical to pre-menstrual symptoms.

Tips for surviving the 2ww

1. *Obsess collectively*

   No matter where you are in your 2ww, there are millions of women the world over at the same stage, having the same highs and lows as you. Luckily, the Internet facilitates communal obsession, so you can share your excitement and anxiety with other people who are at the same stage as you. The Irish websites *www.magicmum.com, www.rollercoaster.ie* and *www.eumom.com* have sections for those TTC, or you can try one of the bigger UK or US sites. There is more information on all of these sites in Chapter 4.

2. *Pamper yourself*

   Go shopping, have a facial or a massage, treat yourself to a night out or a night in – whatever will help you relax and take your mind off the 2ww for a while. The 2ww can become quite stressful if you don't give yourself a break along the way, and only you know what will ease your anxiety for a few hours.

3. *Blog*

   It can be very therapeutic to write down your thoughts and feelings at this stage – whether for your eyes only or for public consumption. Sometimes just working through your feelings about the possibility of being pregnant can help you understand them and cope with them – even if it does make you realise how obsessed you have become! Don't worry, this is normal!

4. *Everything in moderation*

   One dilemma that a lot of women have during the 2ww is whether or not to act as though they are pregnant. Should you eat and drink what you like, and exercise as normal, until you get that positive test, or should you treat your body as being already pregnant? The simple answer is: all things in moderation. A few glasses of wine here and there, a light jog, or a portion of blue cheese will do no damage to a developing embryo. As far as food and drink goes, the placenta is not yet formed, so the embryo is not yet receiving nutrients from your body. You may choose to abstain from your usual indulgences while you are TTC, but it is important to remember that this process may take some time and that you still have to live your life in the meantime.

Time to test

Some people are happy to wait until their period is late before testing. If you are one of those people, please stop reading this section now and skip straight to the next one. You are the lucky women – the ones who will survive the 2ww with the minimum of anxiety. The rest of us want to know if we are pregnant as soon as possible; we are the ones who are in danger of becoming HPT (home pregnancy test) addicts. (OK, I confess, I am already a long-term addict).

The very earliest I have ever heard of anyone getting a second line on an HPT is at 8 DPO. Once implantation has occurred (at 6 to 10 DPO), it takes one to two days for HCG levels to rise enough to be detected by a HPT. So put those tests away for the first half of the 2ww and don't even think about using them.

If you decide to test early (early being before your period is due), then be prepared for a negative test. If you don't see a second line, it will get you down, but try to remember that it can take up until about 14 DPO for your HCG levels to rise to a level that will be detected on a HPT. Promise yourself that if you are going to test early, you won't lose hope until at least 12 DPO.

The dipstick tests that can be bought online (you dip these into a cup of urine instead of peeing on them) are the cheapest and also the most sensitive tests available. They claim to detect HCG at 20iu but they have been known to detect it at 10iu. (I know this because I had a very, very faint line on a test just before a blood test detected a level of 10iu.)

When you test, make sure to follow the manufacturer's instructions. If the test is to be read within ten minutes, then any result that comes up after fifteen to twenty minutes should not be taken as valid. Similarly, any result that comes up within the allotted time but disappears afterwards is still a valid result.

If you do see a line, it can be one of three types. The first is a definite line with definite colour (pink/blue). Congratulations, you are pregnant!

The second type of line is one that is so faint that you're not sure if it's there or if you're imagining it, and you can't quite tell whether the line is white/grey or pink (or blue). This is not a positive result, although it may be the start of a rise in HCG. All you can do is test again the following morning and hope for a darker line.

The third type of line is an evaporation line and can be found on many brands of HPT. As the HPT starts to dry out after thirty to forty-five minutes, you may see a grey or white line in the place where you would expect to see a pink or blue line. This is a negative result and is simply the line where the solution that tests for HCG has been placed on the HPT. This is an evaporation line – or, as I call it, the line where a line should be.

For those who want any further information (and you will), there is a wealth of information – and photographs – about every possible type of HPT and OPK at *www.peeonastick.com.*

Home-pregnancy tests (HPTs) and ovulation-prediction kits (OPKs)

One of the most important pieces of advice I can give you when you start out on your TTC journey is where to buy HPTs and OPKs. You can of course nip out to your local chemist but, at ten quid a pee, you probably won't be doing this on a regular basis. The cheapest and most sensitive tests can be found online for as little as about 30 cent each. The question I always get asked about these is: are they reliable? In my experience, they are 100 percent reliable; the only problem with them is that they are so cheap, they encourage a several-a-day habit.

The cheapest tests I have found online are at *www.saveontests.com.* This is a Canadian site that I have been using for years now, and I have always had an excellent service. The tests usually arrive about a week after I have ordered them.

Another site I have used is *www.testsforless.com.* This US site sells the same tests as *www.saveontests.com* and doesn't charge for postage. It tends to work out a little more expensive but is still great value for money.

If you prefer a site closer to home, *www.accessdiagnostics.co.uk* and *www.medicaltestcentre.ie* both sell tests at huge savings compared to high-street chemists but neither can match the value of the first two sites.

One line or two?

If you have followed all the recommendations for timed intercourse and have still not been successful, don't panic: the most fertile among us still have only a one in five chance of conceiving every month. If you have been having well-timed intercourse for six months or more and have still never seen that second line, it may be worth contacting your GP or gynaecologist, who can arrange some simple preliminary tests. There is more about these in Chapter 5.

The thin pink line

If you are a lucky couple in possession of a positive HPT, then what next? Most people go to their GP to get the pregnancy 'confirmed', but there is no need to do this. All your GP will do is test again with another HPT. You can book your maternity hospital and/or obstetrician yourself; you do not need a referral letter.

If you live in an area where you have a choice of maternity hospital, then the best place to ask about the pros and cons of each is online. *www.magic-mum.com*, *www.rollercoaster.ie* and *www.eumom.com* are three busy Irish websites that cater for mums and mums-to-be. If you ask about a maternity hospital in the Pregnancy section of one of the websites, then you should get enough answers to help you make an informed choice. For those who do not have Internet access or friends and family to ask, here are details of Irish maternity hospitals, so that you can contact each hospital directly with your queries.

REPUBLIC OF IRELAND
Portiuncula Hospital, Ballinasloe, County Galway – (090) 964 8200
Maternity Services, University College Hospital, Galway – ((091) 544 544
St Munchin's Regional Maternity Hospital, Limerick – (061) 327 455
Cork University Maternity Hospital – (021) 492 0500
Tralee General Hospital, County Kerry – (066) 718 4000
St Joseph's Hospital, Clonmel, County Tipperary – (052) 77 000
Mayo General Hospital, Castlebar – (094) 902 1733
Sligo General Hospital, Sligo – (071) 917 1111
Letterkenny General Hospital, County Donegal – (074) 912 5888
Midland Regional Hospital at Mullingar – (044) 934 0221
Midland Regional Hospital at Portlaoise – (057) 862 1364
Our Lady of Lourdes Hospital, Drogheda, County Louth
    – (041) 983 7601
Cavan General Hospital, Cavan – (049) 437 6000
Waterford Regional Hospital, Waterford – (051) 848 000
Wexford General Hospital, Wexford – (053) 915 3000
St Luke's General Hospital, Kilkenny – (056) 778 5000
Rotunda Hospital, Dublin – (01) 873 0700
National Maternity Hospital, Dublin – (01) 637 3100
Coombe Women's Hospital, Dublin – (01) 408 5200
Mount Carmel Hospital, Dublin – (01) 492 2211

NORTHERN IRELAND
Altnagelvin Area Hospital – (028) 7134 5171
Antrim Area Hospital – (028) 9442 4000
Causeway Hospital – (028) 7032 7032

Craigavon Area Hospital – (028) 3861 2898
Downpatrick Maternity Hospital – (028) 4461 3311
Lagan Valley Hospital – (028) 9266 5141
Mid Ulster Hospital, Magherafelt – (028) 7963 1031
Daisy Hill Hospital, Newry – (028) 3083 5000
Erne Hospital, Enniskillen – (028) 6632 4711
Mater Infirmorum, Belfast – (028) 9074 1211
Royal Maternity Hospital, Belfast – (028) 9089 4656
Ulster Hospital, Belfast – (028) 9048 4511

The next choice you have to make is between public, semi-private and private care. Again, you will find a wealth of information online, and it is advisable to get as many opinions and experiences as possible when it comes to making this decision and when deciding which obstetrician to book if you choose to go semi-private or private. Be warned, many obstetricians get booked up very quickly, so you should research this as early as possible.

Finally, if you have Internet access, you should check yourself into a 'birth club'. A birth club is a section of a parenting website that is dedicated to all the mums-to-be who are due in a particular month. You can follow others' pregnancy experiences, as well as sharing your own, as you all go through the ups and downs of the eight-month wait together.

3

Charting your fertility signs

Introduction

Charting your fertility signs simply means keeping track of your waking temperature each morning and making a daily note of your cervical mucous (CM), cervical position (CP) and ovulation prediction kit (OPK)/ovulation monitor result (all of these methods are discussed in Chapter 2) in order to predict your ovulation day. You may choose to keep track of one or more of these fertility signs: the more of them you chart, the more accurate your ovulation prediction will be. It should be noted that these methods can be used to avoid pregnancy as much as they can be used to try and achieve it.

While CM, CP and OPKs can all predict that you are probably about to ovulate (in the next one to three days), the only fertility sign that can tell you that you have definitely ovulated is your basal body temperature (BBT). Your BBT is your body temperature at rest. If you take a reading at the same time and under the same conditions every day, you should see a pattern emerging over the duration of your cycle. During the follicular phase, your temperature should be lower than during the luteal phase. Once you have ovulated, you should see a sustained shift in temperature. This is due to the release of progesterone from the corpus luteum (see Chapter 2), which causes a rise in temperature. These two different levels of temperature create what is known as a biphasic chart. If you are not pregnant, your temperature should dip back to pre-ovulation levels on the day before, or the first day of, menstruation. If you are pregnant, your temperature should stay raised and may even rise to a third level; this is known as a triphasic shift.

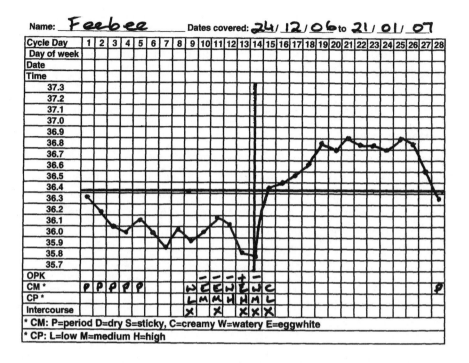

Fig. 3.1 A typical non-pregnant chart

A common reaction to the idea of charting is: 'What a load of hassle, I couldn't be bothered!' If you couldn't be bothered, then you probably haven't started to get frustrated with TTC yet and are happy enough to keep trying in the manner you have been so far. Good luck, and I hope you never need to return to these pages! If you are starting to get fed up with failed cycles, then charting your temperatures and other fertility signs is a good way of maximising your chances of pinpointing ovulation and taking control of your fertility in a way that makes you feel like you are doing something to help yourself. It may also help you recognise whether there are hormonal or other problems with your cycle, and you can then seek help on those grounds if you wish.

The psychological boost that this feeling of control can give you should not be underestimated. Whether you have been TTC for several months or have just begun trying, the fact that you are doing everything that nature allows you to do to help you conceive can save you from the helplessness that can befall all TTCers at any time.

And it's not that much hassle. Really! 'Temping' (taking your temperature) is just a question of reaching for the thermometer when the alarm goes off in the morning. Most digital thermometers retain the last reading, even when they are turned off, so you won't need to record it immediately. So rest assured, you can snooze as long as you like afterwards.

Charting your temperatures

Getting started

The first thing you need is a BBT thermometer that is accurate to two decimal places. This differs from a regular thermometer in that it measures body temperature in hundredths of degrees as opposed to whole degrees or tenths of a degree. You can use either a mercury or a digital thermometer; however, I recommend a digital one, as it is quicker to use, beeps when it has finished recording your temperature, and is far easier to read.

You can buy digital BBT thermometers in Boots for around €19 and from *www.accessdiagnostics.co.uk* for around €14. Lidl and Aldi also do them periodically for about €4: if you keep an eye out on the TTC boards on *www.magicmum.com* and *www.rollercoaster.ie*, you can often see posts from other users advising when they are in stock.

In order to see a definite pattern of ovulation, you need to be consistent about how you take your temperature. Here are some key guidelines to follow when taking your BBT.

Taking your temperature

1. Your BBT needs to be taken after a minimum of three hours of uninterrupted sleep, so the best time is first thing in the morning. Make sure it is the first thing you do, before you go to the toilet or talk on the phone, as any significant movement can result in a change in temperature. If you wake up less than three hours before your usual waking time, then take your temperature and make a note of the time.

2. You need to take your temperature at the same time every morning (within a half-hour timeframe), as your temperature rises gradually throughout the morning, so the later you wake, the higher your temperature will be. If you do wake earlier or later than usual, then make a note of the time.

3. Most people choose to take their temperature orally. You may also take it vaginally, but once you start that way, you should continue

until the end of the cycle, as vaginal temps tend to be higher than oral temps.

4. Make a note of any circumstances (see below) which may contribute to an unusually high or low temp. One or two temps that do not fit with an ovulation pattern are not usually anything to worry about.

5. Take a break from temping for about six days at the start of your cycle. Temps during menstruation and for a couple of days afterwards are not important.

Special temping circumstances

1. *Illness*

   Illness and infections, in particular those that cause fever, can cause your temperature to be significantly different to usual. Also, any drugs or medication that you may need can have a similar effect.

2. *Alcohol*

   Drinking large amounts of alcohol the night before you take your temperature will almost certainly result in a spectacularly high temp the next day. One or two drinks shouldn't have much of an effect, but if your temp is unusually high, then make a note of the previous night's drinking.

3. *Sleep disturbances*

   Insomnia, night-waking and general poor sleep patterns can make charting your temperatures challenging. If you wake more than three hours before your usual waking time and can get back to sleep, then use the temp you record when you wake again. If you wake less than three hours before your usual waking time, take your temperature then and make a note of the time. If you do not manage three hours of uninterrupted sleep during the night, then take your temperature at your usual waking time and make a note of your sleep disturbance. Don't worry too much about your sleep patterns, just do the best you can.

4. *Travelling*

   Travel, even within the same time zone, can cause fluctuations in BBT. This should be limited to the day of travel and the following day. If you are in the luteal phase of your cycle, it should not affect your chart much and you should still see a sustained shift in temperature. However, if you are coming up to ovulation, then you may want to take some simple steps to make sure you identify the day of the thermal shift.

If you are travelling to a time zone an hour or two ahead or behind, you can simply take your temperature an hour or two later or earlier than usual while you are away. If this is not possible, then you can plan in advance. If you are travelling an hour ahead, then try to change your waking time by twenty minutes for the three days prior to travel. You can then do the reverse when you return. This technique can also be employed for changing to Daylight Saving time and back again. If you are travelling long-haul, then it's probably best to stick to your usual waking time in the new time zone and be prepared that your temps may be a little higher or lower than usual for a day or two.

Having said all that, I wouldn't bother with any of it! The worst that can happen is that your temps are a bit too high or too low for a couple of days, and if you're unsure about your ovulation date, well you'll just have to get down to business for an extra night or two (that is if you are travelling with your partner)!

5. *Shift work*

If you work various shifts then you may find that your temps fluctuate a little from day to day. The most important thing is to take your temperature after your longest period of sleep, regardless of what time of day it is. As long as you have had at least three hours of uninterrupted sleep, then you should get an adequate reading. Even with changes in waking time, you should still be able to identify a clear thermal shift during your cycle.

One or two unusual temperatures during your cycle should make little difference to your ability to identify a pattern of ovulation on your chart. If these temperatures happen around ovulation time, then make sure you pay extra attention to your other fertility signs, so you still have a fairly good idea of when ovulation has occurred.

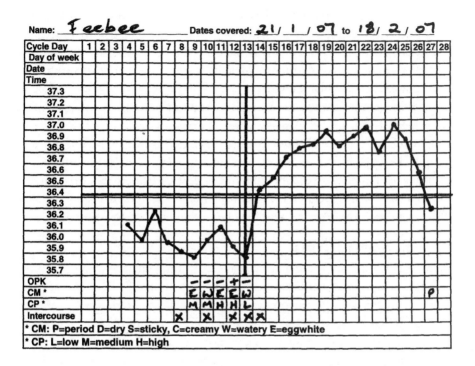

Fig. 3.2 A typical chart

Typical chart features explained

This is a fairly typical (there is no such thing as typical) non-pregnant chart. The dots mark the BBT for each day and the line connecting them is the temperature curve. The vertical line notes the likely day of ovulation and the horizontal line is known as the coverline. This is an arbitrary line drawn to separate pre-ovulatory (follicular phase) from post-ovulatory (luteal phase) temps and does not really hold any other significance. The hope is that luteal-phase temps will not dip below the coverline before menstruation is expected, but this can happen under certain circumstances and is not necessarily a reason for too much concern.

You can see that there are two very distinct temperature phases, and that the second phase begins shortly after ovulation. Your temperature will not rise until you have ovulated, as the temp rise is triggered by the release of progesterone from the corpus luteum (see Chapter 2), and this happens after the egg has been released from the follicle. However, although most people will see a temp rise the day after ovulation, it can take up to three days. You can see that temps begin to fall towards the end of the luteal phase, and in this case, the temp falls below the coverline on the first day of menstruation.

There is also an area below the temperature curve to record your other fertility signs, should you wish. The exact terminology you use will depend on how you choose to record your fertility signs. You can create your own chart, photocopy the blank chart at the end of this chapter, or use online or downloadable software that does most of the calculations for you (more on this later).

CM refers to cervical mucous; this can be recorded on this chart as P (period), D (dry), S (sticky), C (creamy), W (watery) or E (egg-white). CP is cervical position and is recorded here as L (low), M (medium) or H (high). You can also mark incidents of sexual intercourse, positive and negative OPKs, and any other factors that may be of importance to your chart.

Different chart patterns

There's really no such thing as a typical chart. Most charts deviate from the textbook sample to a certain extent, and there shouldn't be any reason to worry about this as long as you can discern a sustained temperature shift in the second half of your cycle. Likewise, not all of your fertility signs will necessarily indicate ovulation on the same day: you should allow up to a three-day margin of error for each fertility sign. So you may have a positive OPK one day, followed by fertile CM the next day, followed by a temperature rise two days later. Ovulation is likely to have taken place on the third day, although it could also have happened the previous day, or even the day before that.

There are also some further chart patterns that you may or may not experience. Some women will see these patterns on their chart once or regularly; many will never note them.

1. *Low temperature before ovulation*

   Some women experience a lower than usual temp the day before
   ovulation, alerting them to the fact that ovulation is imminent. This
   is thought to be due to the effect of the LH surge that triggers ovulation (see Chapter 2). Not all women experience this, though, and
   even those that do, do not see this on every cycle. I get this sometimes; sometimes I don't.

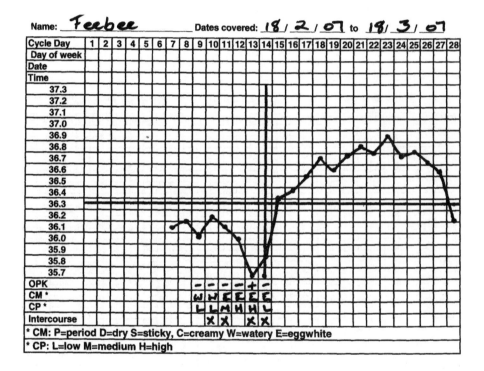

Fig. 3.3 Chart with a low temperature before ovulation

2. *Fallback temps*

Sometimes you may see a temperature rise in the few days after ovulation, only to have a much lower temp at 3 or 4 DPO. This happens when oestrogen, which can lower your temperature, is still present in sufficient amounts after ovulation. You may also notice some fertile-quality CM around this time. This usually only happens for a day or two at most, and you should expect to see your temp rise to post-ovulation levels again afterwards. This is something that I have experienced on several cycles, including one pregnant cycle, so don't panic if your temp drops suddenly in the early stage of your luteal phase.

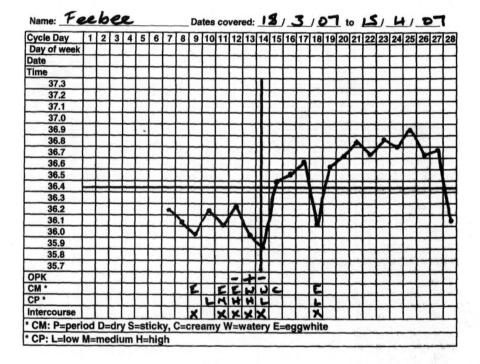

Fig. 3.4 Chart with a fallback temp

3. *Implantation dip*

The term 'implantation dip' is used to refer to a dip in the temperature curve that can take place during the expected time of implantation (if pregnancy has occurred), which is usually between seven and ten days after ovulation (7 to 10 DPO). The dip is usually just one low temp amongst the higher luteal-phase temps. It is thought to happen because the corpus luteum peaks in its progesterone production around this time. If conception does not occur, then the corpus luteum starts to recede. However, if a fertilised egg starts to implant in the uterine lining, then the corpus luteum is prompted to keep producing progesterone in order to support the pregnancy until the placenta can take over hormone production. The dip in temperature happens as the embryo is implanting and before the corpus luteum has been alerted to keep going.

A dip in temps around the time implantation is expected to take place does not necessarily mean that you are pregnant. This is a pattern that is also seen on non-pregnant charts. One of the reasons given for this is an unexpected yet not uncommon surge in oestrogen during the luteal phase, which can lower temps for a day or two.

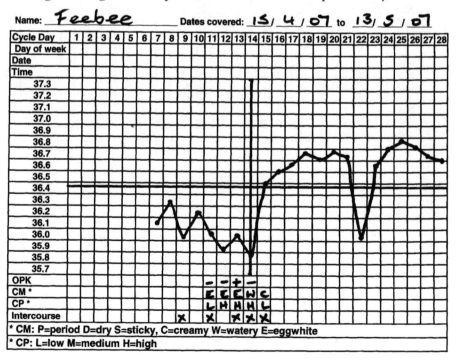

Fig. 3.5 Chart with an implantation dip

4. *Triphasic chart*

A triphasic chart shows three levels of temperatures: pre-ovulation temps, post-ovulation temps, and then a third and even higher level of temps towards the end of the luteal phase. It is often said that triphasic charts are more likely to indicate pregnancy, but this pattern can be seen on non-pregnant charts with the same frequency.

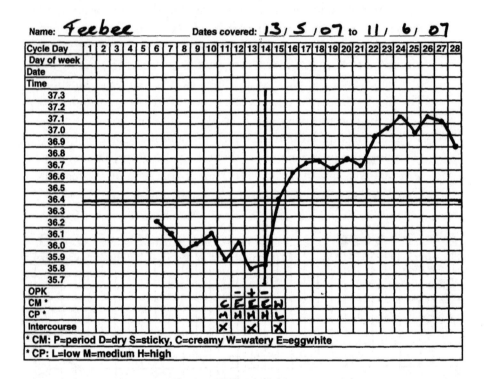

Fig. 3.6 A triphasic chart

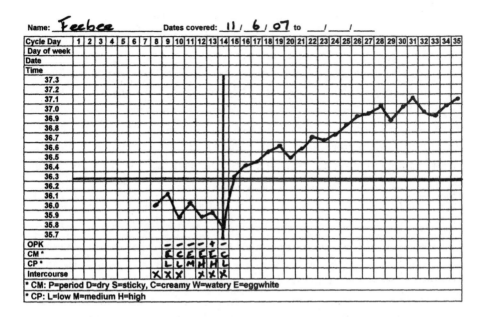

Fig. 3.7 A pregnant chart

The only difference between a pregnant and a non-pregnant chart is that you will generally not see a temp dip towards the end of the luteal phase if you are pregnant. Temps should stay elevated beyond your usual luteal-phase length, and it is recommended that if this happens you should take a home pregnancy test. Of course, in the real world you have probably taken several by that stage. Very few people wait the full two weeks before testing, especially those who are committed enough to be charting in the first place. (If you are one of those that are able to wait it out, then good for you: don't be sucked in like the rest of us!) However, it is still possible (though unlikely) that your HCG levels may not be high enough for a positive test, even at 14 DPO, and continued high temps at this stage may still indicate pregnancy.

You may also continue to get high temps, even after your period has arrived: it once happened to me that my temps didn't fall until the second day of my period. It is also possible that your temps might fall towards the end of your luteal phase and you may still be pregnant. Both of these situations are unlikely but do sometimes happen.

Recording your fertility signs

You can record your fertility signs very easily and accurately by simply putting pen to paper. This may be the easiest thing for you if you just want to wake up, take your temp, make a note of it and be done with it for the day. You can keep your chart beside your bed and mark your temp on it as soon as you've taken it. The Boots BBT thermometer comes with a book of blank charts for this purpose. Alternatively, you can photocopy the blank chart at the end of this chapter or create your own chart to suit your needs. There are also some digital alternatives, which can make charting easier and more fun.

Fertility Friend

www.fertilityfriend.com is the home of the Internet's most popular charting software. It is an American website but the terminology is universal so there are no language barriers. Fertility Friend is free to join and membership includes access to its basic charting software. VIP membership, which gives you more charting features and access to the busy message boards, is $10 per month, $16.95 for ninety days or $45 for a year. All the functionality you really need to chart your fertility signs is contained in the free membership, and the VIP membership is only really useful if you want to participate in the message boards. It is still great value, though, as you will find all the info you will ever need to know about charting and fertility from other FF members, not to mention the support that is on offer from others in the same boat.

The charting software itself is very easy to use. You simply click on the relevant date on the calendar, enter your BBT, the time you took it and any other relevant info. Almost all possibilities are covered by drop-down menus and tick boxes, and if there is an event you want to record that is not already covered, you can create your own tick box or enter it in the notes section. The software then works out, based on all the information you have given, when you are in your fertile phase, when ovulation is likely to have taken place, and where your coverline should be drawn. Over time, it also adds in statistical information it has gathered from your previous cycles.

Once you have been charting for a few cycles, you will probably have no problem working out your fertile phase, ovulation day and coverline yourself. However, it is still reassuring to have FF confirm this. There may also be times when you disagree with FF's assessment: maybe you have had a fallback temp and/or fertile CM after ovulation, and the day this happened has been reassessed as your ovulation day when you are sure you ovulated a couple of days previously. If you are sure of your own judgement, then feel free to ignore FF's assessment. For a second opinion, just post a link to your chart on one of the message boards: you are bound to get some educated feedback.

There is also a wealth of information on the site in the form of articles and tutorials, and user-generated facilities such as a chart gallery and HPT and OPK galleries. One warning though: using the site can become addictive!

Taking Charge of Your Fertility

Taking Charge of Your Fertility (TCOYF), available at *www.ovusoft.com*, is a downloadable software program that has much the same features as the Fertility Friend software. The main difference between the two is that you must be online to use FF, whereas once you have downloaded TCOYF you can use it on your own computer, even if you are not connected to the Internet. TCOYF is available to download for free for a fifteen-day trial; after that, it costs $39.99. The website also offers free message boards, where you can discuss all aspects of fertility and the software itself.

The functionality of the software is similar to FF in that you can choose a date from a calendar and enter your details for that day; TCOYF then creates a chart for you. The chart indicates periods of low fertility, high fertility and infertility, and works out your likely ovulation date once you have got to that stage in your cycle. The software has a Help function that contains information on fertility, charting and using the software itself. Any other answers you need, you should get on the website's message boards.

Identifying problems on your chart

Whichever method you use to record your fertility signs, you should be able to build up an accurate picture over a short number of cycles. Most women won't have a perfect, textbook chart, and cycles can vary from month to month, but you should be able to identify a clear shift in temperature around midway in your cycle. If you are having problems seeing a biphasic pattern, or if ovulation is not happening when you expect it to, it can be cause for concern. Some of the reasons for a less than picture-perfect chart are listed below, but if you have real concerns about your cycles you should get a full hormone profile done by your doctor. There is more information about this in Chapter 5.

1. *Short follicular phase*

   The main reason for a shorter than usual follicular phase (less than twelve days) is a higher level of the follicle-stimulating hormone (FSH). Once a woman reaches her late thirties (and before that in many cases), it becomes increasingly difficult for her body to mature the follicles in her ovaries in preparation for an egg to be released. To compensate for this, higher levels of FSH are produced by the pituitary gland, the follicles mature more quickly, and the egg is released sooner. An increase in FSH levels is not reversible, so if you suspect that this may be a problem for you, get your FSH levels checked on day 2 or 3 of your cycle as soon as possible. Your doctor can then decide on a course of action to help you conceive, as high FSH levels are generally associated with lower fertility. There is more information on this in Chapter 6.

   Another cause of early ovulation may be fertility drugs that you have taken in the previous cycle. Although most fertility drugs should be out of your system by now, anecdotal evidence suggests that the effects can sometimes be enough to stimulate egg production in a subsequent cycle.

2. *Long follicular phase*

   Many women may not ovulate until day 20 or 21 of their cycle, and if this is normal for you, then it is not anything to worry about. A longer than usual follicular phase, whether it be an increase from twelve to fourteen days or from twenty to thirty days, can be caused by a number of factors. Both physical and psychological stress can have an effect on the body and can delay ovulation. Illness, travel, exercise and weight gain or loss can also have the same effect. A longer than usual follicular phase may affect only one cycle or it can disrupt a number of consecutive cycles if the cause is ongoing.

3. *Short luteal phase*

Much has been made of a short luteal phase (LP) or a luteal phase defect (LPD) on the Internet. This usually refers to an LP of less than ten days. Many online resources will tell you that an LP of eight or nine days is insufficient for implantation to occur. I don't agree with this and feel that it is only a problem if there is an underlying hormonal issue. One possible cause of a short LP is insufficient progesterone production, usually caused by a poor quality of ovulation. Progesterone deficiency can indeed cause problems with implantation if the corpus luteum does not produce enough progesterone to sustain a pregnancy.

Your GP, gynaecologist or fertility specialist can take blood to check your progesterone levels at 7 DPO to make sure you are producing sufficient progesterone. The test results will also tell you if you have produced enough progesterone that cycle to have ovulated, but you will probably already be able to tell that from your chart. If you are ovulating but your progesterone levels are low, this may be helped by progesterone supplements, which should be taken from ovulation, and also by taking Clomid in the follicular phase to improve the quality of ovulation. However, with Clomid it is advisable to have ultrasound monitoring in the run-up to ovulation, as this medication can cause multiple eggs to be produced, which in turn can result in a high-risk multiple pregnancy.

4. *Long luteal phase*

It is unusual to see a luteal phase of longer than sixteen or seventeen days unless pregnancy has occurred. If yours is longer than this and you are definitely not pregnant, then it is advisable to see your doctor.

5. *Anovulatory cycle*

It is not uncommon to have a single cycle over a period of time where you do not ovulate. You may also have a bleed at the end of this cycle, as normal, and if you are not charting, you may not have any reason to believe that you did not ovulate. An anovulatory cycle can be caused by the same factors that cause delayed ovulation: stress, illness, travel, exercise and significant change in weight. There are also periods of a woman's life where she may not ovulate regularly or at all. These include adolescence, pregnancy and while breastfeeding.

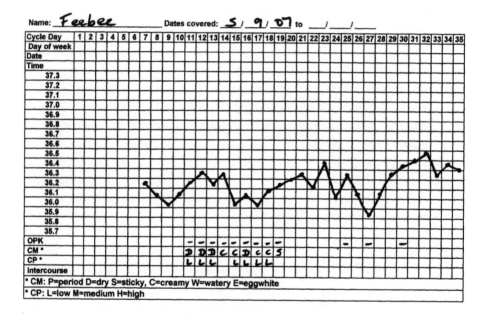

Fig. 3.8 An anovulatory chart

The above are all temporary causes of anovulation, however. There are also a variety of medical conditions that can cause women to stop ovulating indefinitely. These include elevated prolactin levels and other pituitary-gland problems, as well as polycystic ovarian syndrome (PCOS). There is more information on the causes, diagnoses and treatments of these conditions in Chapter 6.

Sinead from Waterford

Of all the TTC courses of action to take, this is the cheapest, and probably what you should do first if you have reasonably regular cycles. You can get the thermometer in Boots for about €20 and download blanks charts from the Internet.

I didn't want to temp because it was another symptom of TTC taking over my life, as you have to take your temp first thing in the morning. It was my acupuncturist who asked me to do it. And now, after a year, it is like second nature to me. At the start, I would fret if I forgot to take it, but now I'm not that bothered if I miss a day or two – which, funnily enough, is usually at the weekend. I find *www.fertilityfriend.com* a really good website for tracking all the information.

Another benefit of temping is that you don't have to buy HPTs because you can see near the end of your cycle, if your temp drops, that your period is on the way – at least that's how it is for me. In fact, I don't have the dreaded 2WW; it's only a 1WW for me. I can see that there is no change in my pattern and so can stop hoping for the last week.

I am now doing my first IVF, and am still temping.

However you decide to record and chart your fertility signs, you should find it a rewarding process. You will learn a little more about your body, about your cycles and about your ovulatory patterns. When you have been TTC for a while, you can feel as though you have surrendered control of a significant part of your life. Charting can help you feel you are taking back a little of that control, and helping the process along in some small way. And, of course, the knowledge you gain from it may turn out to be invaluable.

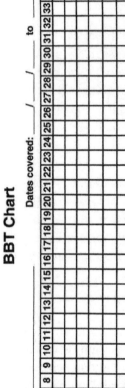

Fig. 3.9 A blank chart for you to copy and use

4

The Internet: from AF to BFP

Introduction

The Internet is the first port of call for many people who are looking for information and support to help them through their TTC journey. There is a wealth of information on every conceivable aspect of fertility available online, and there are also men and women all over the world going through the same processes, the same highs and lows as you, and looking for others with whom they can share their experiences.

While some couples may tell friends and family that they are trying for a baby, most are unlikely to share the intimate details. However, TTC can be a very thought-consuming process, and many women (and some men) are eager to talk to others who are in the same situation. Internet support groups can offer a means of sharing experiences, getting answers, pooling resources and making friends. Whether you are just starting out on your journey and looking for information or are seeking emotional support to help you through infertility, there are like-minded, non-judgemental people out there who have the same hopes and dreams as you.

Getting started on the Internet

If you have not yet ventured online, or if you don't feel confident about finding your way around, then a good starting point is Alex French's book *DOT ie: A Practical Guide to Using the Internet in Ireland*. This book covers the basics of getting online, Web browsing and email, online travel and shopping, message boards and chat rooms, and viruses.

Looking for information online

Whatever your question, the Internet has an answer. There is no guarantee that it is an accurate or reliable answer, though, so you need to know where to look and whom to ask. The more knowledgeable you are about using the tools of the Internet, the more likely you are to benefit from the results.

Search engines

A search engine, such as Google (*www.google.com*) or Yahoo! (*www.yahoo.com*), is a program that searches pages on the Web for specific key words and returns a list of all relevant results. So if you want to find information on how to identify your fertile days, then type 'identify fertile days' into your search engine. This search will give you in excess of a million results. While you will probably find plenty of advice that will help you pinpoint your fertile days, there is no guarantee that the web page you have chosen to view contains accurate or up-to-date information. Search engines will give you quantity but not necessarily quality.

If you are specifically looking for medical information, then you can try a medical search engine, such as Search Medica (*www.searchmedica.co.uk*) or Web MD (*www.webmd.com*). This will filter out a considerable amount of the results that may show up on a general search engine, and should provide you with information that is more relevant to your enquiry.

Before embarking on a course of action prescribed to you by a search engine, you need to be sure that the information has come from a trustworthy source. If the website is familiar, e.g. the BBC News site or the VHI site, then the information will probably be accurate. If you do not recognise the provider, then you may want to get a second or third opinion.

Finally, make sure you don't become a cyberchondriac! The Internet has given us the power to self-diagnose certain conditions, but it also has the potential to cause widespread alarm amongst those looking for answers. If you are looking for information on breast pain and you land on a site about cancer, move swiftly on. If your period has been uncharacteristically light this month, do not worry yourself sick because 'Dr Google' tells you that this is a symptom of menopause. If you are genuinely worried about a pain in your breast or an unusual development in your menstrual cycle, then you should take your concerns directly to your GP.

Fertility websites

The best place to start looking for general information on having a baby is a fertility or TTC website, or a parenting website with a TTC section. You can use a search engine to look for one, or you can try any of those reviewed in this chapter. Many websites have their own search facility, so you can try to find information directly or you can browse the site for topics of interest.

Many parenting or TTC websites also have communities you can join to share your experiences with others. Participation in these communities is usually organised through a message board, which facilitates many-to-many communication. Numerous websites also have blogs, which allow one person to communicate to many readers, and those readers to post their views on the topic of discussion. Message boards and blogs are discussed in more detail in this chapter.

The type of TTC website that suits you best may well depend on how long you have been trying for a baby. If you are just starting out, then a parenting website with a TTC section may be an ideal solution, as you will expect to move from the TTC to the parenting section before long. That way, once you find a website that you enjoy, you can stay for the long haul.

However, if you have been at this game for a while, then you may prefer a fertility website where you won't be bumping into other people's pregnancies and babies on a regular basis. Fertility Friend (*www.fertilityfriend.com*) is an excellent site with informative articles, communities for every stage of the process, and software for charting your cycles. (There is more on this in Chapter 3.) It is a US-based site, so if you would prefer something more local, you could try *www.irishinfertilitysupportforums.ie.*

Most pregnancy and parenting websites started life without much advice on getting pregnant in the first place. However, most have found that their message boards are inhabited by a large amount of TTCers, and so have developed TTC and fertility sections to give advice and support to the many users who need it.

Seeking help from others

No matter where you are on your TTC journey, there are others out there at the same stage. Whether you are looking to share your emotional experiences or the details of any physical problems you may have encountered, there is a message board or a blog that will allow you to share your thoughts with like-minded people. It may also help you to find information on procedures you have not yet considered.

In the past, those having problems TTC had to rely for support and information on people close to them, most of whom would have had no experience of fertility problems. In some cases, a lack of understanding can be more alienating than no support at all. The popularity of message boards and blogs as support networks means that you don't have to go through the depression and trauma of infertility alone.

Message boards

An Internet message board, or bulletin board or forum, is an application that allows users to post messages and hold discussions online. The forum may allow anonymous messages or may require users to register in order to participate. Internet message boards are an excellent source of information, as users regularly share their own personal stories or advice they have received from their doctors or other health-care practitioners. Most message boards have a search facility which allow you to find discussions on a certain topic.

Internet message boards also have another very important function: they can be an invaluable source of support. Message boards allow you to find others in similar situations with whom you can chat and swap stories. Whether you have just started TTC and are looking for advice, or have been trying for a while and want someone to talk to, there is a message board out there for you.

Again, you can find these through search engines and through parenting and fertility websites, or you can try some of the boards listed in this chapter. It's a good idea to 'lurk' a little first (view posts without posting yourself), to get to know the tone and temperament of other users before you commit yourself. It's important to find an environment in which you feel comfortable, so you can get the support and feedback that you need. Some message boards thrive on debate and confrontation, whereas others may foster an environment where differing viewpoints are not always welcome. It's up to you to find one that suits your personality and TTC requirements – keeping in mind that you might not always get on with every other member!

Most TTC communities provide a wonderful support network for those trying for a baby, but it is important to remember that one size does not always fit all. If you have recently set out on your TTC journey, then you will probably want to share your first flush of enthusiasm and excitement with like-minded TTCers. On the other hand, if you have been trying for some time, you will probably need support from others in the same boat. Most message boards have sections for different stages of the process, and also cater for those who may need specific procedures or treatment in order to conceive. You may also find sections for those trying for the second or third time, or those who have suffered a loss. You might also want to consider whether you would prefer a busy US or UK board, where you can remain completely anonymous, or an Irish board, where you can get local information or meet up with others, should you wish to.

Once you have invested emotionally in a message board, you may begin to feel a real sense of community with other users. It is likely that most of you are at the same stage of TTC. Some, maybe most, of those people will go on to become pregnant; hopefully you will be one of them. But what if you're not? What if you have to face one pregnancy announcement after another, until your brave face becomes too hard to wear?

Once it becomes too painful to remain part of a group, leave. Join a more suitable group if you want. When you are sharing your experiences of TTC with others, you have to be prepared for the fact that they may become pregnant before you. When you are starting out, this may give you hope, but if you are the person who has been left behind more than once, then it can be a painful experience. If it is too hard for you to remain in contact with a person or a group, do what is right for you and move on. Don't worry about your friend: she is pregnant!

Irish TTC websites

www.makingbabies.ie

This is my own site; it features advice on TTC, information about this book, and the blog I have been writing since my first miscarriage.

www.vhi.ie

The VHI site has a reasonable amount of up-to-date articles on fertility, infertility and miscarriage. The best way to access these is to do a search within the site, or to use their Health A-Z directory. There is also a busy message-board area, with a Pre-pregnancy section for TTC and infertility advice and information.

www.rollercoaster.ie

Rollercoaster is a pregnancy and parenting website with very little information on fertility. It does, however, have busy message boards where you can find advice and information on TTC, infertility, pregnancy loss and adoption and fostering.

www.eumom.ie

EUMom is another pregnancy and parenting website with a limited amount of articles and a busy message board. There is no board dedicated to TTC, although there is a busy TTC thread on their Miscellaneous board.

www.magicmum.com

Magic Mum is a message board, pure and simple. It is predominantly pregnancy- and parenting-based, although there are also a large number of general sections. There is also a busy TTC board, a TTC With Assistance board, a Pregnancy Loss board and an Adoption board. In my opinion, Magic Mum is the parenting message board that fosters the best sense of community, and it is easy to navigate and search.

www.irishinfertilitysupportforums.ie

This is Ireland's first website dedicated to infertility, set up by Helen Quinn, who has been there, done that. Like Magic Mum, it is solely a message board and, again like Magic Mum, it has a great sense of community.

www.alternativeparents.com

Alternative Parents Ireland is an information site for lesbian, gay, bisexual or transgendered couples and singles who have, or are planning to have, children. There is information on fertility, self-insemination and artificial-reproduction techniques.

UK and US TTC websites

www.mumsnet.com

MumsNet is a UK pregnancy and parenting site with a very active message board. There are no articles on fertility but a search of the site will bring up all the fertility-related threads from the message boards.

www.babycentre.co.uk / www.babycenter.com

Baby Centre/Center is a pregnancy and parenting site that also has a Getting Pregnant section, with advice on fertility and TTC. There are also message boards for TTC and fertility problems.

www.mothering.com

Mothering is first and foremost a US parenting site but has a good stock of articles on fertility, which are best accessed through the site's search function. There is also an active Fertility board on the Mothering Dot Commune forum.

www.parenthood.com

Parenthood.com, a US-based site, has a comprehensive Conception section on its main website and a busy Conception message board that deals with different areas of TTC.

Linda from Dublin

I found Internet message boards to be a great support because, although there might be someone around you going through something similar, for many people infertility is a private battle, and going online affords some degree of anonymity. The first time I did IVF I used a forum based in the UK (*www.iVillage.com*). I didn't even know there was an Irish board! While it was great to have the support there, I have to say I find it much better being able to talk on an Irish board (*www.magicmum.com*) to people attending the same clinic as me. It's brilliant to be able to ask questions about the medications, clinic personnel, appointment waiting times, and so on, and get an informed opinion.

I used to have a signature on Magic Mum that included a picture of my little boys in it but I took it out because I was posting on the infertility board so often, and I was afraid some might think it insensitive. Also, [my partner] Robert was concerned that someone from 'real life' would identify the boys and know then that they were IVF. I always wonder, though, what you do if you bump into someone from the Internet in the clinic waiting room! It's a small forum I'm in now, and everyone is aware of when people's appointments are, so you can't help looking about the room and wondering 'Is that X?' I suppose it's easy to think of Internet groups as a virtual world, but Ireland is such a small place that it doesn't have the anonymity of boards in larger countries. Of course, this can be good or bad, depending on your point of view!

Blogs

A blog (short for 'web log') is an online journal on any subject imaginable. Most blogs are created using software that allows the blog's owner to submit a post, which then appears on the blog's web page as the most recent journal entry. Most blogs allow readers to comment on the blog post's content, and so debate and friendships begin. Many blogs also contain links to other blogs with similar content, and this is how a network of friendship and support can build up.

Blogs can provide insight into a person's life or a particular situation in their life. Readers can offer their own advice and share their experiences. Some blogs, in particular those that tell a story, can become addictive, as readers come back daily to see how the plot unfolds. This is often true of TTC blogs, as everyone wants to see a happy ending. There are some fantastic infertility blogs out there, and the quality of some of the writing never fails to amaze me. I suppose people who are used to fielding thoughtless comments from others are bound to choose their words carefully – although the level of humour in most of them is a pleasant antidote to the sadness of the situation.

TTC blogs

Here are a few to get you started. All link to several other great blogs, so you can have a look around and find the ones that appeal to you.

2weekwait.blogspot.com
    My own personal journey.

www.tertia.org
    After being so close for so long, I have finally arrived. Life after infertility.

www.alittlepregnant.com
    Madcap adventures in infertility, pregnancy and parenthood.

stirrup-queens.blogspot.com/2006/06/whole-lot-of-blogging-brought-to-you.html
    Big list of blogs.

Setting up a blog could hardly be easier. Most blogging software is designed to make writing blog posts as easy as writing an email. Some blogging software is free; other facilities are available for a small monthly fee. Some of the more popular sites for setting up your own blog are listed below.

Blogging software

www.blogger.com

Blogger is a free blog-publishing service.

www.livejournal.com

Livejournal is an online community which offers members free blogging software.

www.wordpress.com

Wordpress is a open-source blog-publishing system that offers both a free and a subscription service. Wordpress also offers a large number of plug-ins and features.

www.typepad.com

Typepad is a subscription blog publishing system with many additional features, which is aimed at non-technical users.

Once you've set up a blog, you must remember that you are publishing to the world, and libel laws apply. Make sure that everything you write about other people is factual and not open to interpretation. You should also keep an eye on any comments you receive, as you will be responsible for monitoring the content. You may also have the misfortune to have a troll visit you. The most important thing to remember with trolls is . . . don't feed the troll! If someone posts an inflammatory comment on your blog, the best thing you can do is ignore it or delete it. Trying to explain yourself to someone who is insistent in winding you up can only end in frustration for you. Also, given the nature of infertility blogs, you may receive comments from people who just don't get it and may end up upsetting you. Again, you do not need to reply, but if you do, you should keep it brief and polite: some people will never get it. However, these occurrences have been few and far between for me, and the good of blogging has always easily outweighed the bad.

Why do I blog? I blog because it gives me an outlet for the pain and frustration of infertility, and because it lets me explain my feelings without interruption. I blog because writing my experiences in a coherent manner makes me feel better about myself. I blog to let people know the reality of infertility. I let people know about my blog because letting them read about our struggles is easier than having to explain them face-to-face, and it allows them to keep up with our news without having to ask me constantly. It also allows them to decide when is a good time to call and when I might prefer to be left on my own. I consider my blog an achievement, something positive that has come from our infertility.

Privacy and the Internet

Whether or not you intend to remain anonymous when posting on a message board or writing a blog, it is important to consider certain privacy issues before you begin. You would be surprised how easy it is to identify someone from a few harmless pieces of information, especially in a such a small pond as Ireland. I have recognised a poster on a TTC board by a simple piece of information that gave away no personal details. We worked together, so I was one of the few people in real life who was privy to that particular piece of information. We are now friends, so that story did have a happy ending. I have recognised several other people from snippets of information they have posted online. Some I have contacted; some I have left alone.

There is nothing wrong with being up front about who you are and what you're going through. I do not mind if people recognise me online, as my struggle is a part of who I am and I am happy for people in real life to know what we have been through. Not everyone is in a position to be that open, though, especially if they feel that it could impact on their work life or their personal relationships.

Guarding your privacy

The best way to protect your privacy is to choose a username that does not identify you in any way, and preferably one that you have not used in the past. It is important to remember that message-board posts are generally archived and therefore remain in circulation as long as the message board exists. So everything you post on any message board will be accessible to everyone on the Internet for an undetermined length of time. If you have used a partic- ular username in the past, then a quick Google search of that name could bring up posts on another forum, and you may not have been so guarded about your identity before.

If you have to register on a site or message board, don't use your real name or your work email. Don't put specific details in your profile. If you wish to share these details with other users, then you can use the private-mes- saging facility on the message board.

You should also consider the nature of the information you are sharing and whether it may have implications for the future. For example, you may feel comfortable telling people that you are going for a test, but what if the results are not what you expected, and not the sort of information you want to share? Your online friends (and lurkers) may deduce from your silence that something is wrong. Most people will be genuinely concerned and support- ive about your plight; you are all in the same boat and have the same goal –

a baby. However, don't forget that anything you post is available to anyone with an Internet connection, so it is possible that your boss, your parents or your neighbours may stumble across your news.

Fertility websites

www.fertilityfriend.com

Fertility Friend's main purpose is to provide online software to help women chart their menstrual cycles (see Chapter 3). Limited (although adequate) use of the software is free, and more features are available for a small membership fee. This also gives users access to the extensive message boards, which provide information and support for all stages of the TTC process. There are also plenty of articles that explain all aspects of fertility. A must for anyone who is serious about taking control of their fertility.

www.ovusoft.com

Ovusoft provides downloadable software for charting your cycle. This is available as a trial and can then be purchased. There is also a busy message board for support and guidance.

www.peeonastick.com

Everything you ever needed to know about home pregnancy tests (HPTs) and ovulation prediction kits (OPKs).

Infertility websites

www.infertilityireland.ie

Infertility Ireland is the website of the National Infertility Support and Information Group. There is not a huge amount of information available online but they do organise regional support meetings, so it is a good starting point if you would like to meet other couples suffering from infertility.

www.irishinfertilitysupportforums.ie

This is Ireland's first website dedicated to infertility, set up by Helen Quinn, who has been there, done that. It is a message board and has a great sense of community.

www.fertilityzone.co.uk

Fertility Zone is an excellent UK message board that covers all areas of fertility treatments and loss.

www.fertilityfriends.co.uk

Fertility Friends is an extensive UK message board with regional boards and also sections where you can ask questions of medical professionals.

www.infertileworld.co.uk

This is a sister site of *www.fertilityfriends.co.uk*, containing news and articles on infertility.

www.inciid.org

The International Council on Infertility Information Dissemination is a US-based organisation with news, articles and insight from medical professionals available on its website.

www.resolve.org

Resolve is the US national infertility association. The website offers a wealth of information and articles written by people in the know. A great resource for help and advice for dealing with issues surrounding infertility.

www.ivfconnections.com

IVF Connections has an extensive message board for those undergoing IVF. There are sections for every possible circumstance and message boards for people in different parts of the world.

Val from Waterford

Without Internet message boards, I would have had a much harder time dealing with our infertility. I found I was not alone: we weren't the only couple experiencing the sadness, anger, self-doubt and hopelessness you go through on your journey. The boards are also a fantastic source of information from people who have been through it all, who can steer you in the right direction and give you all the information you were anxious to discover as you started out on your journey.

They are also a fantastic means of venting your emotions: many people don't want to be bothering friends and family all the time with their highs and lows, and feel they have to bottle everything up. I've often turned to a message board to simply get it all off my chest, rather than bend the ear of a friend or family member, who I fear may be tired of listening to my constant trials and tribulations. Without fail, other posters have responded with words of support or empathy, and we can all feel a little better, having talked it out amongst people who are experiencing the same frustrations and upsets as we are.

I've personally made some wonderful friends through message boards; I've met like-minded women who I 'clicked' with, and would now count them among my best 'real-life' friends. We meet up for coffee and a chat, swap stories, and generally do all the things that friends tend to do together.

In today's world, people are often disconnected slightly from friends and family due to the transient nature of living: maybe you moved away from your homeplace, or perhaps you have a long commute to and from work, leaving little time for friends, or family gatherings. The pressures of modern life impinge on our private time, and our support networks, and Internet message boards go some way to providing an instant connection with like-minded people who are willing to reach out and support others. The best thing is that they're always there, no matter where in the world you are; at the click of a button, a whole community is ready to help you make sense of it all.

Learn the lingo

Once you have braved the TTC message boards and blogs, you will notice straight away that a lot of acronyms are used. These may be new to you, but don't despair, you will be speaking TTC before you know it! Here are some of the more commonly used abbreviations:

2ww	Two Week Wait, the wait between ovulation and testing
AF	Aunt Flo, your period
BBT	Basal Body Temperature
BD	Baby Dance, intercourse (also DTD, see below)
BFN	Big Fat Negative, pregnancy test
BFP	Big Fat Positive, pregnancy test
CD	Cycle Day
CF	Cervical Fluid (also CM)
CL	Coverline
CM	Cervical Mucous (also CF)
CP	Cervical Position
DH/DP	Dear Husband/Partner
DF	Dear Fiancé/Fiancée
DS/DD	Dear Son/Daughter
DPO	Days Past Ovulation
DTD	Do The Deed, intercourse (also BD)
EDD	Estimated Due Date
EWCM	Egg-white cervical mucus
FSH	Follicle-Stimulating Hormone
GnRH	Gonadotropin-Releasing Hormone
HCG	Human Chorionic Gonadotropin, hormone detected by pregnancy tests
HPT	Home Pregnancy Test
IUI	Intra-Uterine Insemination
IVF	In-Vitro Fertilisation
LH	Luteinising Hormone
LMP	Last Menstrual Period, the first day of your last period

LP	Luteal Phase
LPD	Luteal Phase Defect
MC, M/C	Miscarriage
O	Ovulation
OPK	Ovulation Prediction Kit
PG	Pregnant
POAS	Pee On A Stick
TTC	Try(ing) To Conceive

Here are some general Internet abbreviations that you may also come across:

AFAIK	As Far As I Know
BTW	By The Way
FAQ	Frequently Asked Questions
FWIW	For What It's Worth
FYI	For Your Information
IRL	In Real Life
HTH	Hope This Helps
IMHO	In My Humble Opinion
IMO	In My Opinion
LOL	Laugh Out Loud
ROTFL	Roll On The Floor Laughing

5

When nature is not enough

Introduction

If you've been having well-timed intercourse for several months and have never seen that second line, you might start to wonder if it is ever going to happen. TTC can be a stressful occupation, and it is normal to feel anxious after three or four months if you have had no success. Three or four months is not a particularly long time to be TTC but it is a large chunk of your year that has been dedicated to trying, hoping, praying for a baby. Some couples can carry on their lives as normal while TTC, but others put everything on hold in anticipation of that positive pregnancy test. So how do you know when it is time for you to look for help?

The human fecundity rate

The human fecundity rate (the probability of achieving a pregnancy in any given cycle) for fertile couples is about 20 percent. That means that 20 percent of couples will conceive on their first cycle, 16 percent on their second and 13 percent on their third; after twelve months, only 7 percent of couples will still be trying. To put it another way, if you took a hundred couples with no known fertility problems, you could expect twenty to be pregnant after a month, thirty-six after two months and forty-nine after three months; after a year, ninety-three should be pregnant.

Months TTC	Percentage of fertile couples who will conceive that month (to one decimal place)	Number of fertile couples (out of 100) who will be pregnant by the end of that month
1	20	20
2	16	36
3	12.8	49
4	10.2	59
5	8.2	67
6	6.6	74
7	5.2	79
8	4.2	83
9	3.4	87
10	2.7	89
11	2.1	91
12	1.7	93

So there is only about a one in five chance that you will conceive on any given cycle, even if you have no fertility problems. If you have not conceived after three or four months, then try not to worry: you are most likely just one of the slow starters.

On the other hand, however reassuring these statistics might be, they show nothing of the emotional impact of TTC and how difficult a whole year of trying can be. They are also of little comfort if you are one of the 17 percent of couples (one in six) who will need medical assistance to have a baby.

When to look for help

So how do you know which category you fall into and when it is time to seek help? The definition of infertility varies from country to country but is generally considered to include those couples under thirty-five who have been having well-timed intercourse for a year and those over thirty-five who have been trying for six months.

However, a year is a long time to wait if you are not having any periods, are having irregular or painful ones, or simply find it too hard to deal with the immense disappointment that comes at the end of every month. Also, if you waited a year to see a doctor, and then were told that you had sperm problems or were not ovulating, you would probably wish that you'd sought help sooner.

It is really up to you to decide when is the right time to step on to the rollercoaster of investigations and treatment. If you've reached the one-year milestone but are happy to keep trying on your own, then don't feel pressured into having tests and procedures. If you've been trying for six months and are finding things very difficult, or have reason to believe that there may be a problem, then don't wait any longer just because you've been told that you have to keep trying for a year.

Where to turn for help

Your GP

The first port of call for most couples who are having difficulty conceiving is their GP. Your GP can conduct some simple, non-invasive tests and can then refer you to a fertility clinic for further investigations if necessary. This is something you can do while continuing to try on your own, and if the test results show any problems, you can move swiftly on to a specialist, who will offer you further tests and treatment.

However, some people have reported that their GP was reluctant or unwilling to take any of these steps unless the couple had been trying for at least a year. My advice, should you come up against this obstacle and really want some answers, is to lie. Just a little white one. If you have been trying for eight months and you just can't face another failed cycle, or you feel there is something wrong, then nobody will be any the wiser if you tell them that you have been trying for a full twelve months.

I am not trying to subvert the Irish medical system here, I am just suggesting a little intervention to combat the fact that the emotional side of fertility problems is rarely addressed amongst the medical profession. A year is a very long time to keep getting your hopes up and having them dashed, and then trying to pick yourself up to start all over again. And if you have a problem (such as low sperm count or anovulatory cycles) that can be identified by a simple blood test or semen analysis, then the sooner your problem is discovered, the better.

If you have been charting your temperature or your fertility signs, or both, bring your data along with you to your appointment. It may not mean that much to your GP, but if he or she is familiar with fertility issues, it may help in pinpointing a potential problem.

Your gynaecologist

Your gynaecologist will be more familiar with fertility issues than your GP, so if you have attended a gynaecologist or obstetrician in the past, you may prefer to contact them first. Your gynaecologist will be able to carry out the same simple tests as your GP and will be in a better position to suggest a course of action if the results show a problem. For example, if your blood-test results indicate that you are not ovulating, your gynaecologist can prescribe drugs to deal with this. If your problem is beyond the scope of your gynaecologist, you should ask to be referred to a fertility clinic.

Again, bring along your charts and fertility data, as they may help your gynaecologist identify a problem. It will also indicate that you are familiar with your menstrual cycle and with basic fertility terms and issues.

Don't be fobbed off

I hear regular reports of couples being told at a first appointment that they have plenty of time and should go off and keep trying on their own for another six months or a year. If you have psyched yourself up for tests and are prepared to move forward with treatment if necessary, then don't let yourself be fobbed off, no matter how young you are. Young people suffer the monthly disappointment just as much as older ones! And you can go off and keep trying on your own forever, but if you have a problem such as blocked tubes, you are never going to get pregnant without help.

If your GP or gynaecologist is reluctant to help you, then find another one. Ask on Internet message boards for GPs in your area who have a good understanding of fertility issues. There is no reason why a couple in search of help shouldn't be given some basic tests. The cost and stress of such tests is negligible in comparison to the emotional cost of having to keep trying for another six months or a year when you are already desperate enough to contact a medical professional.

Of course I am not suggesting that you shouldn't listen to your GP or gynaecologist: they are the experts and will strive to do the best for you. However, time and again I see how the emotional side of TTC and infertility is neglected in favour of practical medical concerns. A GP who suggests that a twenty-five-year-old couple should try for another year, in an effort to spare them the stress of fertility treatment, may not be aware that the stress of TTC for more than a year can become too much for some couples.

Online support

The Internet is a great source of support and information (see Chapter 4). If you are a regular user, then this may be the first place you go when you need advice. Here you can enquire as to what to ask your GP or gynaecologist, what sort of experiences people have had at the various fertility clinics and what to expect when you embark on the road of fertility treatment. If you are having problems, you can ask advice and read about other people's experiences.

However, try not to be too swayed by strong personalities and anecdotal evidence. In the end, your medical practitioner is the person who knows the best course of action for you and will help you achieve your dream. If you don't get on with your doctor for some reason (and a clash of personalities can happen in all relationships), then find a doctor whom you trust, and allow him or her to guide you.

Jane from Dublin

As soon as we were married, I threw away the birth-control pills with glee. I was probably a little naive but I was also full of confidence, so we threw ourselves into the 'baby-making' with gusto! A year went by and nothing was happening. I bought countless books and read various articles and websites about what we should and shouldn't be doing. I was taking folic acid, hubby was taking zinc, and we bought a fertility monitor to help us along. But still no luck, and I was eventually referred to a gynaecologist by my GP. The gynaecologist took one look at us and our history and practically laughed us out of the room. He said that women read too much these days, and 'in the old days' women wouldn't even get to see a doctor until they'd been trying for two or three years. He discharged us and told us to come back in a year if nothing had happened by then. His parting words were along the lines of 'Sure you're only thirty-three, you've plenty of time'. I was distraught after that appointment. I cried and cried when we got home. I was so frustrated that, after sixteen cycles, we were still being told to just relax and it'd happen. I felt as though I was being treated like a hysterical and foolish woman who should pull herself together.

Six months later, I decided to go and see another gynaecologist, and this one talked to me like the intelligent woman I hope I am. He didn't use platitudes or sympathy; he talked statistics and results. He was clear that after our twenty-two months trying, it was time for us to start treatment, and we agreed a regime of drugs and follicle tracking. Finally, I felt relief that I was being taken seriously, that we were finally moving forward in our quest, and that there was hope again. For so long I had been living with the constant, repetitive highs and lows of my cycles, and now finally someone was going to help us do something about the problem. I'm still terrified that we may not have a baby, but at least we're doing something other than 'just relaxing'!

Systematic investigations

There are four basic tests that should be conducted on any couple seeking help to have a baby. The tests are mostly non-invasive (although the HSG can be uncomfortable and even a little painful) and should either diagnose or rule out a large number of conditions. Sperm problems, ovulation problems, hormone-related issues, diminished ovarian reserve, uterine abnormalities and blocked tubes can all be at least indicated, if not diagnosed, by the four basic tests outlined below.

1   Day 3 and 7DPO blood tests

Blood tests carried out at specific times during a woman's menstrual cycle can determine whether or not her hormone levels are within the normal range. These are usually done on day 3 (but can be done on day 2 if necessary) of the menstrual cycle and at about seven days after ovulation. The main hormones that are checked on day 3 are FSH (follicle-stimulating hormone), LH (luteinising hormone) and E2 (oestradiol – a form of oestrogen). The levels of these hormones can start to change by day 4 of the menstrual cycle, so it is important to get a measure of where they are before this happens.

FSH is secreted by the pituitary gland and stimulates the ovaries to mature follicles in preparation for ovulation. An elevated level on day 3 indicates that the brain is having to work harder to stimulate the ovaries; this is likely to be a sign of a diminished ovarian reserve. This means that the egg supply is reducing at a greater rate than normal and can be a cause of infertility (see Chapter 6). It also means that fertility drugs are likely to have less of an effect than on those women whose FSH lies within the normal range.

E2 levels can be closely linked to FSH: if FSH is within the normal range but E2 is abnormally high, this can mean that the FSH level has been artificially suppressed. If this happens, it is advisable to have the tests repeated.

The LH level should be similar to the FSH level. If it is higher, this can be an indication of PCOS (see Chapter 6). Other non-cycle-specific hormone tests that can be carried out at this time are TSH (thyroid-stimulating hormone) and prolactin, both of which can have an effect on the menstrual cycle, and thus on fertility.

The table below gives details on the range of hormone levels and an explanation of the values:

HORMONE	NORMAL VALUES	EXPLANATION OF VALUES
FSH	3 to 20mIU/ml	In general, a level of 3 to 6 is excellent, 6 to 9 is good, 9 to 10 is fair, 10 to 13 suggests diminished reserve, and 13 to 20 is very poor. Over 20 tends to mean perimenopause.
E2	92 to 275 pmol/l	Abnormally high levels may indicate a diminished ovarian reserve or a cyst.
LH	<7 mIU/ml	A level that is higher than the FSH level may indicate PCOS.
TSH	0.4 to 4 mIU/ml	A high level generally indicates hyperthyroidism, which can affect fertility.
Prolactin	<24 ng/ml	A high level can indicate hyperprolactinaemia, which can affect fertility.

DAY 3 HORMONE LEVELS

A further blood test at seven days past ovulation (7 DPO) can be done to check whether or not ovulation has occurred. This test checks progesterone levels: a level of 10–15 ng/ml indicates that ovulation has occurred and that the corpus luteum is producing progesterone (see Chapter 2). However, some doctors prefer to see higher levels to ensure that you are producing enough progesterone to sustain a pregnancy, and may suggest progesterone supplements for your next cycle.

It is important that this test is done on the correct day of your cycle. It is sometimes called the day 21 blood test, on the assumption that every woman ovulates on day 14 of her cycle. If you rely on this assumption, however, your test results may not be accurate. If you have actually ovulated on day 20 of your cycle, there is no point in having the test the next day: you will have to wait until day 27. If you know when you have ovulated, make sure to schedule your test for seven days later.

2   Semen analysis

A semen analysis is a simple test that checks for the number of sperm present in a sample (sperm count), the percentage of sperm that can move forward normally (sperm motility) and the percentage of sperm that are normally shaped (sperm morphology). The analysis also usually includes tests for antisperm antibodies and white blood cells. The semen sample can be procured at home and brought to your doctor within an hour, or you can collect it at your doctor's office, whichever you prefer.

Below is a list of the normal range of values for the various sperm parameters and an explanation of each value. There is further information on all of this in Chapter 6.

PARAMETER	NORMAL VALUES	EXPLANATION OF VALUES
Count	≥ 20 million/ml	Between 10 and 20 million sperm/ml is considered low, and below 10 million is very low.
Motility	≥ 50 percent Grade A or B	Motility is graded from A to D. Less than 50 percent Grade A or B is considered low.
Morphology	≥ 15 percent normally shaped	Less than 15 percent normally shaped sperm is considered low.

SEMEN-ANALYSIS PARAMETERS

As the quality and quantity of sperm can change from month to month, a follow-up test should be conducted about six weeks after the first test.

Home test fertility kits

There are some tests on the market that allow you to check your own FSH level and sperm quantity and quality at home. The home sperm test kits are available from *www.accessdiagnostics.co.uk* for £19.99 for two tests, and the FSH tests are available from the same site for £5.99 for two tests. They are also available from Boots for €120 for both tests.

3   Post-coital test

Some doctors recommend a post-coital test as well as a semen analysis, in order to check that the sperm move normally in the woman's cervical mucous. The test involves the collection of the cervical mucous within two to eight hours of the couple having sex. The test is usually done one to two days before ovulation, when the cervical mucous is thin, stretchy, plentiful and best suited for transporting sperm. If you are tracking your fertility signs, you will have a good idea when you are coming up to ovulation. If not, your doctor will probably advise you to keep an eye on your cervical mucous or to use an ovulation-prediction test, which gives you between twelve and seventy-two hours' notice that ovulation is about to happen (see Chapter 2).

4   HSG (hysterosalpingogram)

A HSG is an X-ray examination during which dye is injected through the cervix and into the uterine cavity. It is used to check whether or not the fallopian tubes are open. If they are open, the dye flows through the tubes and spills out into the abdominal cavity. A series of X-rays are taken during this procedure in order to document the flow of the dye and help with the diagnosis. The X-rays can also be used to check for certain uterine abnormalities, but these are usually diagnosed by a further procedure called a laparoscopy (more on this in Chapter 6). The procedure takes about ten minutes and is not usually painful, although some women report pain and cramping when the cervix is opened in order to inject the dye. A couple of strong painkillers about a half hour before the procedure should be enough to ensure that it is not too uncomfortable. You may also experience some cramping afterwards.

What next?

If your initial tests show up a problem, and it is something that is outside the expertise of your GP or gynaecologist, you will be referred to a fertility clinic. If your test results come back normal and you wish to proceed with further tests and investigations, you should ask to be referred to a clinic. Most clinics require a referral letter but they will generally allow you to book an appointment and then organise the referral letter. You should call your local clinic for clarification on this issue. The Sims Clinic in Dublin allows patients to self-refer: in other words, you don't need a referral letter but can just go ahead and book an appointment yourself. The Morehampton Clinic also allows self-referral, but their treatment is limited to IUI with donor sperm.

You should also talk to your GP/gynaecologist and each of the clinics in your area before deciding where to go. Not all clinics offer all fertility treatments, waiting lists can vary considerably from clinic to clinic, and some clinics offer public and medical-card treatment, whereas others do not. You may also wish to ask about clinics and consultants on message boards in order to find the one that is most suitable for you.

Irish fertility clinics and contact details

CLINIC	TELEPHONE	WEB	REFERRAL
Sims Clinic Rosemount Hall Dundrum Road Dublin 14	(1800) 49 77 77	*www.simsclinic.ie*	None needed
Merrion Fertility Clinic 20 Holles Street Dublin 2	(01) 678 8688	*www.merrionfertility.ie*	Referral needed
HARI Unit Rotunda Hospital Parnell Square Dublin 1	(01) 807 2732	*www.hari.ie*	Referral needed
Clane Hospital Prosperous Road Clane County Kildare	(045) 982 300	*www.clanehospital.ie*	Referral needed
Kilkenny Clinic Green's Hill Kilkenny	(056) 775 1420	*www.thekilkenny clinic.com*	Referral needed in some cases
Galway Fertility Unit University Hospital Galway University Road Galway	(091) 544223	No website	Referral needed
Cork Fertility Centre Fernhurst House College Road Cork	(021) 4865764	No website	Referral needed
Morehampton Clinic 136 Morehampton Road Donnybrook Dublin 4	(01) 2839463	*www.infertility.ie*	None needed

Dealing with waiting periods

One of the most difficult things to deal with when you start on the road to fertility treatment is the amount of waiting that you have to do. First of all, you have to wait for test results, which can take a couple of weeks. Then you may have to wait several months for an appointment at a fertility clinic. Then there's more waiting for further procedures, review appointments with your doctor, mandatory blood tests, and then simply getting in the queue for treatment. For me, it took nine months from the time my gynaecologist referred me to a clinic to when I started my first IUI. I called my blog 'The Waiting Game', as it seemed as though that was all I was ever doing.

The first thing you should do is to prepare yourselves for a long wait. If there is more than one fertility clinic in your area, then it's worth calling around to find out which has the shortest waiting list, as these vary all the time. You can also put yourself on the clinic's cancellation list: there tends to be a significant drop-out rate, as people do become pregnant naturally while waiting for treatment. I got cancellation appointments at both clinics I attended several months earlier than my original appointment. I don't like waiting!

Secondly, try not to build yourself up too much for each appointment. At times, I would focus so much on the date of my next appointment that I would begin to imagine that all our problems would be solved on that day. Just take each consultation or test as a step towards your goal, and not the goal in itself.

Finally, give yourselves something to look forward to during the long wait. If your next appointment is not for three months, book a night out or a weekend away for the six-week mark. That way you have something else with which to pace yourself.

Joanna from Dublin

I shouldn't have had any problems. I had a child. I was only thirty-four. I was having plenty of sex. So where was the baby? I had been charting, and timing intercourse; I figured there was something up and went to my gynaecologist after only seven months.

In fairness to my gynaecologist, he took me very seriously from our first visit and had a plan of action in place for me straight away. He suggested three rounds of Clomid and, if nothing was shaking at that stage, he proposed a post-coital test, followed by a laparoscopy. Before any tests or treatment had begun, I became pregnant and miscarried. My doctor decided there was no need for tests, as the sperm were obviously getting to where they needed to be.

But after four cycles of Clomid, including a cycle that spanned Christmas – my second disappointing Christmas, at this stage – I was exhausted from the whole ordeal and desperately depressed. At my very next appointment, I asked what next, and my gynaecologist suggested injectable meds. This was the big guns, and so he would be transferring me on to a fertility clinic.

Things started to get frustrating. Having become comfortable with my doctor, who was progressive and knew me, I was thrown back to the beginning, with unfamiliar procedures and doctors who didn't see me at all.

I faced horrendous red tape and frustrating waits, as I was told 'You need this test or that before proceeding, so it'll be next month, not this month, before you go on', or suchlike. I needed my CD3 bloods to be taken again, and given that I was on day 5, I was too late! Frustration! Then I was told I should have an HSG before going on, despite my gynaecologist assuring me I didn't need one. Why didn't they take his word for it! I was allowed to proceed in the end without one, but only after a big fight. Why do they make you fight, when all your fight is used up against your own body, against infertility? I eventually got the go-ahead to proceed to a medicated cycle of IUI, and was completely hyped to do it, when they found a cyst at my baseline scan. Devastated again, and another wait.

The next cycle went better, and I got to do an IUI. I had a chemical pregnancy from this, and was both encouraged and devastated.

I was now up to two years' trying, and nothing happening. I'd had enough of fighting and switched to a different clinic. I wish I'd done it sooner. My appointment was in October, I had my bloods tested within a week, and my IVF cycle started at the end of December. Pregnant. Success. The end.

Alternative therapies

Some of you may wish to explore alternatives to Western medicine, either as a complement to the treatment you are getting from your GP, gynaecologist or fertility doctor, or because you wish to pursue more natural, holistic practices.

Traditional Chinese Medicine

Traditional Chinese Medicine (TCM), which includes acupuncture, herbs and changes to diet and lifestyle, has been shown to have positive effects on fertility. In particular, acupuncture has been shown in scientific studies to increase pregnancy rates with IVF.

TCM looks at broadly the same problems and deficiencies as Western medicine – hormone factors, ovulatory function, sperm problems – but rather than supplementing deficiencies with medication, it looks at correcting the function that is creating the deficiencies in the first place. TCM, as a holistic approach to fertility, is not a quick fix and is something that you will need to do over a number of cycles to see any progress. Many people do acupuncture in conjunction with Western fertility treatments, and your fertility clinic may offer this as a supplemental procedure.

However, if you choose to stick exclusively to Western approaches, it is still worth considering acupuncture if you are doing IVF. As I mentioned, studies have shown that acupuncture an hour or two before embryo transfer increases pregnancy rates. This is probably because acupuncture helps regulate the autonomic nervous system (involved in the control of muscles and glands), which helps make the lining of the uterus more receptive. The same theory applies to having acupuncture around the day of expected implantation for natural cycles.

Other alternative therapies

While there is little evidence to suggest that aromatherapy, reflexology, massage therapy or hypnotherapy can directly help infertility, they can all help alleviate some of the stress that infertility causes. And of course, they do no harm.

Financial considerations

Fertility treatment is costly, and the actual procedures (IUI, IVF, ICSI) are not covered by any Irish medical-insurance company. I have spoken to Bertie Ahern personally about this and he has told me that he will 'look into it'. I look forward to his report.

Furthermore, fertility treatment is not offered on the public health service. The HARI Unit at the Rotunda in Dublin runs a public clinic, but the waiting list is a lot longer than for the private one. The Merrion Fertility Clinic in Dublin and the Galway Fertility Unit at the University Hospital offer a discount to patients who hold medical cards. The Cork Fertility Centre offers IVF to medical-card patients under certain circumstances, but each case is decided on a discretionary basis.

Consultations, blood tests and other investigations (such as scans, hystersalpingograms (HSGs) and laparoscopies) should be covered by health insurance, but check with your insurance provider first.

The real savings with Irish fertility treatment come thanks to the government's Drugs Payment Scheme (see *www.citizensinformation.ie*). The DPS allows individuals and families to limit the amount they spend on approved prescribed drugs, medicines and appliances to €90 per calendar month. So no matter how many fertility drugs you need, you will never pay more than €90 euro for them in any calendar month. This amounts to savings of thousands of euro in many cases.

6

Defining infertility

Introduction

The definition of infertility varies from country to country but generally refers to those couples who have not been able to get pregnant after one year of trying, or after six months of trying if the woman is over thirty-five. It can also include those couples who have not been able to carry a baby to term. Infertility affects one in six couples and is something that involves both members of a couple, regardless of where the physical problem lies. Apart from the fact that the emotional impact of infertility hits both partners, investigations and treatments will involve both of you at various steps along the way.

Infertility is an umbrella term for the many different conditions that make it difficult, and sometimes impossible, for a couple to achieve or maintain a pregnancy. These conditions can be identifiable, such as blocked fallopian tubes or low sperm count, or can fall into the category of 'unexplained infertility', the medical profession's way of saying that they just haven't worked out the problem yet. Female problems account for approximately 35 percent of infertility cases, male problems account for about 35 percent of cases, 20 percent involve a combination of both, and about 10 percent are unexplained.

This chapter takes you through some of the more common causes of infertility in order to help you understand what may be going on in your, or your partner's, body. You may also find it helpful to talk to others in the same boat: contact details for relevant support groups are included in each section. If you wish to talk to others online, you should be able to find support groups for each condition on many of the websites detailed in Chapter 4.

While the information contained in this chapter and elsewhere may help you to understand the different conditions involved, it is essential that you contact your GP, gynaecologist or fertility specialist in order to obtain an accurate diagnosis and treatment plan. For more information on taking this step, see Chapter 5.

Common medical conditions – for women

Endometriosis

What is it?

Endometriosis is a condition where tissue similar to that found in the lining of the uterus is found elsewhere in the body. Endometriosis tissue is most commonly found inside the pelvis, around the ovaries, in the fallopian tubes, on the outside of the uterus, or in the area between the rectum and the uterus, known as the Pouch of Douglas. It can also be found in caesarean-section scars, in laparoscopy scars, and on the bladder, bowels, vagina, intestines, colon, appendix and rectum. In rare cases, it has been found in other parts of the body, such as the skin, eyes, spine, lungs and brain. It is important to note that endometriosis is not an infection and is not contagious.

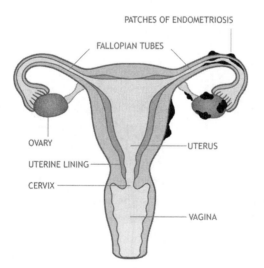

Fig. 6.1 Endometriosis

Every month, as your body goes through the hormonal changes of your menstrual cycle, the oestrogen secreted by the maturing follicles in your ovaries causes the uterine lining to build up. If a fertilised egg does not implant in this lining, then the lining will break down and bleed. The blood is then released from your body as a period. Endometriosis tissue reacts to the secretion of oestrogen in the same way: it grows, it breaks down and then it bleeds. However, this internal bleeding has no way of leaving the body. This leads to inflammation, pain and the formation of scar tissue, known as adhesions.

Endometriosis can be a chronic and debilitating condition and can cause chronic pain, fatigue, lack of energy, depression, sexual problems and, of course, infertility. It is not known why some women develop endometriosis and others do not. It is estimated that 30 to 40 percent of women with endometriosis are infertile.

What are the symptoms?

The most common symptom of endometriosis is pelvic pain. This is most common before, during or after menstruation and during ovulation, but can happen at any stage of the menstrual cycle. You may also experience pain in the bowel during menstruation, when passing urine, during or after sexual intercourse, and in the lower-back region. The amount of endometriosis does not always correlate to the amount of pain you may experience; the location of the endometriosis is a greater indicator of pain.

Other symptoms may include diarrhoea or constipation, especially during menstruation, abdominal bloating (again, in connection with menstruation) heavy or irregular bleeding and fatigue and lack of energy.

How is it diagnosed?

The only way to diagnose endometriosis is by a procedure known as a laparoscopy. This is usually done under general anaesthetic. Firstly, the abdomen is injected with gas in order to push the abdominal wall away from the organs so that the surgeon can see them properly. Then a small cut is made in the abdominal wall and the laparoscope (a microscope with a light on the end) is passed through it into the abdomen. The images picked up by the laparoscope are displayed on a monitor, allowing the surgeon to navigate the abdominal region in search of endometriosis.

A laparoscopy is usually done as a day procedure. You can discuss with your surgeon beforehand whether or not you would like any endometriosis found during a laparoscopy to be treated immediately. If you choose to do this, it could mean a longer stay in hospital.

How can it be treated?

Currently, there is no cure for endometriosis. Tissue can be removed but there is no guarantee that it will not grow back. Treatment is designed to reduce the severity of symptoms, improve quality of life and aid fertility.

Removal of endometriosis tissue is also done under general anaesthetic. An incision is made in the abdominal wall and instruments are inserted either to cut and remove the tissue or to destroy it with a laser beam or electric current.

Pregnancy rates are highest in the six to eighteen months following surgery. You should consult your doctor to see if any additional fertility treatment may be necessary to help you conceive.

Alternative therapies

Some endometriosis sufferers report successful pain management through the use of acupuncture and Chinese herbs. The acupuncture points and herbs used in the treatment of endometriosis are chosen to help move blood, break up stagnation and therefore stop pain. The idea is that acupuncture promotes blood circulation and regulates the endocrine system.

Nina Liu of Melt in Temple Bar in Dublin says that she needs to see a woman's medical diagnosis before deciding on a specific treatment. She recommends that the couple don't TTC for at least three months so that she can rebalance the woman's body, help the blood flow, and reduce the endometriosis. She says that endometriosis can be treated with acupuncture and herbs alone but that it is a long process and that many women prefer to have tissue removed by surgery in conjunction with acupuncture.

Support

The Endometriosis Association of Ireland, Carmichael Centre, North Brunswick Street, Dublin 7. (01) 873-5702. *www.endo.ie.*
www.irishinfertilitysupportforums.ie

Polycystic ovarian syndrome (PCOS)

What is it?

At the start of each menstrual cycle, follicles begin to grow in the ovaries. Eggs start to mature in these follicles, and as the cycle progresses one will become dominant and will eventually be released into the fallopian tube during ovulation, while the others disintegrate. With polycystic ovaries, the ovaries are larger than normal and contain a series of undeveloped follicles or cysts. Polycystic ovaries do not necessarily cause any problems, and the condition may not even affect your fertility.

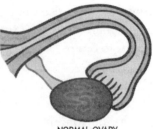

NORMAL OVARY

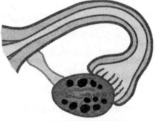

POLYCYSTIC OVARY

Fig. 6.2 Polycystic ovary

Problems arise when the cysts cause a hormonal imbalance and a pattern of symptoms tends to arise. This hormone or endocrine syndrome is known as PCOS. So you can have polycystic ovaries without having PCOS; most women with PCOS also have polycystic ovaries, however.

In PCOS, the ovaries tend to produce an excess of androgens (hormones such as testosterone, which control the development of masculine characteristics), and this can result in a lack of regular ovulation, along with other symptoms. Because of this, PCOS is the leading cause of infertility in women. PCOS affects an estimated 5 to 10 percent of all women of childbearing age. However, many of those are not aware that they have the condition, as all the symptoms do not present in all cases. It can be treated by medication, changes in diet, exercise and acupuncture, but is not curable.

It is unclear what causes PCOS but it does seem to be hereditary to a certain extent. PCOS sufferers often have problems with insulin levels, and some researchers believe that this may cause the excessive production of androgens, which in turn cause PCOS symptoms.

What are the symptoms?

Some women with PCOS have normal, regular periods, but most have some changes to their menstrual cycles. Sometimes bleeding can be very heavy, but it can also be lighter than usual. Periods may be irregular and can also stop completely, resulting in infertility due to anovulation.

Other symptoms include an increase in body or facial hair (hirsutism) due to the excess of androgens, acne, thinning or loss of hair (alopecia), and weight gain and trouble losing weight. PCOS sufferers may also experience patches of dark skin (acanthosis nigricans) on the back of the neck or in other places. This is caused by higher levels of insulin in the blood, which is one of the hormonal changes that can occur with PCOS.

Because of the nature of the symptoms of PCOS, sufferers are more at risk for obesity, diabetes, high blood pressure and heart disease, so it is important that treatment is tailored to the individual needs of the PCOS patient.

How is it diagnosed?

PCOS is generally diagnosed on the basis of the clinical signs and symptoms outlined above. Once your doctor has gone through your menstrual history and symptoms with you, he or she will want to rule out other illnesses with similar symptoms, such as hypothyroidism, elevated prolactin levels, or tumours of the ovary and adrenal glands. You will most likely have a blood test to check your hormone levels and blood sugar. This may be followed up by an ultrasound to check for polycystic ovaries. When all of these things have been considered, a diagnosis is then made.

How can it be treated?

Treatment of PCOS depends to some extent on the woman's stage of life. For those who are not TTC, the birth-control pill can help regulate hormone levels and therefore menstruation. If you suffer from acne or hirsutism, a water pill (diuretic) called spironolactone may be prescribed to help reverse these problems. Spironolactone can have an effect on blood potassium levels and kidney function, so occasional blood tests are needed to check these. Hair loss can be stopped by a medicine called propecia, which blocks the effect of male hormones on hair growth. Both spironolactone and propecia are not recommended during pregnancy and should be stopped before beginning TTC.

For those who experience anovulation and wish to TTC, a medication called clomiphene (usually known by its brand name, Clomid) can be used to induce ovulation. There is a risk that multiple eggs may be released, which can result in twins or triplets (or even more)! Therefore it is advisable for your doctor to perform an ultrasound prior to ovulation, to make sure that you don't have too many dominant follicles.

Metformin (also known by its brand name, Glucophage) is a medication used to treat type 2 diabetes. Because it affects the action of insulin on the body, it can also be used to treat PCOS.

Alternative treatments

Many women with PCOS use multiple medications to help with their symptoms. While these can be helpful, the range of side effects can take their toll. Many women have turned to acupuncture, either as an alternative or as an addition to Western medication. Acupuncture has been shown to have a reasonable degree of success (one study showed a 38 percent regular ovulation rate after three months of acupuncture) in women with low to moderate symptoms, although success has not been proven for those women with high testosterone and insulin levels and for those who are obese.

Acupuncture works by balancing hormone levels and thereby regulating the menstrual cycle. It has also been shown to aid in weight loss. Acupuncturist Nina Liu says that PCOS is by far the most common infertility problem that she deals with. She usually prescribes a programme of acupuncture and Chinese herbs for three to six months. Most clients will start to ovulate after about three months.

Support

The PCOS Association of Ireland, The Carmichael Centre for Voluntary Groups, North Brunswick Street, Dublin 7; (087) 202 3910; *www.pcos.ie*.

www.soulcysters.com

www.irishinfertilitysupportforums.ie

Helen from Limerick

I began my journey at thirty-two, when I was diagnosed with PCOS. I always knew deep down that there was something 'not quite right', as I had amenorrhoea (lack of periods). Even on my wedding day, I figured that I would have difficulty in conceiving, and that the family that we hoped for would not be easy to achieve.

When I was diagnosed with PCOS, I knew nothing about it, but thanks to the Internet I discovered websites devoted to this syndrome. I always had weight issues and still do. There is no actual cure for PCOS, but the symptoms, which can include weight gain, being hirsute, skin tags, and the inability to ovulate can be controlled with diet and medication. PCOS is a very misunderstood and frustrating syndrome. Women are often told to lose weight and that this will 'cure' them, but that in itself is difficult, as losing weight is a very slow battle. For me, infertility was the hardest aspect to cope with.

While I attended Galway University Clinic, we had timed cycles, but to no avail. In 2002, we moved to Cork Fertility Clinic. We began our first IVF/ICSI on 23 June 2003, the day after my mother died. It was a trying time for me. Unfortunately it did not work, and we both felt very raw and bereft, but did not give up. I asked to be put on Glucophage or Metformin, which my doctor was reluctant to prescribe, but I persevered and I found that it did help with a gradual slow weight loss. In 2004, we did two IVF cycles – one failed, and one had to be abandoned as I did not respond to the medication.

Before our IVF journey commenced, Tony and I were offered the opportunity to participate in an RTÉ documentary on IVF entitled 'Making Babies', and this was aired in 2004. At the end of 2004, both Tony and I felt we had had enough, and I was adamant that I would not try IVF again. It was a drain on us both financially and mentally. However, we decided to have one last go, and on 4 June 2005 I discovered I was pregnant in my thirty-eighth year. Finally, on 31 January 2006, after a seven-year journey, our daughter Rowena was born.

I am, and still consider myself to be, an 'infertile' woman, but thanks to the advances in assisted human reproductive technology, Tony and I became lucky with our darling little daughter Rowena, who has changed our lives in ways too wonderful to measure.

Other ovulation problems

About 70 percent of women with ovulation problems have hormonal imbalances related to PCOS. The other 30 percent include women with other hormonal imbalances and those with lifestyle issues, such as stress and rapid weight change, that can affect ovulation. Also, women who have had cancer treatment or those who are coming to the end of their reproductive lives (this can happen prematurely in one's twenties or thirties) can have ovulation problems. This is related to a reduction in (and eventually an end to) the egg supply. This problem is discussed in the next section.

Hormone imbalances

Hormone imbalances can often be traced back to the glands that produce the hormones involved in regulating the menstrual cycle. These glands are the pituitary, the hypothalamus and the thyroid gland. These glands are part of the body's endocrine system and release hormones that control bodily functions, including the menstrual cycle. The pituitary gland, which is located in the brain, secretes LH (luteinising hormone) and FSH (follicle-stimulating hormone), which control ovulation. Any interference with this can cause a lack of, or a poor quality of, ovulation. It also produces prolactin, which can affect other hormone levels, which in turn can affect ovulation. The hypothalamus, also located in the brain, secretes hormones that start and stop the release of pituitary hormones. It can be affected by stress, illness, some medications, and other lifestyle issues (discussed later). Blood tests carried out on the second or third day of the menstrual cycle can assess the function of the hypothalamus and pituitary glands. These tests are discussed in more detail in Chapter 5.

The thyroid is a small gland inside the neck which controls the body's metabolism. If the thyroid produces too little thyroid hormone (hypothyroidism), this can result in the pituitary producing excessive levels of prolactin, which interferes with ovulation. This can be treated with thyroid-hormone-replacement medication.

Even if you are ovulating every cycle, hormone imbalances may still prevent you becoming pregnant. This is because a poor quality of ovulation, where an inadequate amount of hormones is produced, can affect implantation and even result in miscarriage. When ovulation occurs, the follicle from which the egg was released becomes the corpus luteum and produces progesterone. This progesterone plays a vital role in converting the lining of the uterus into a form that will allow the implantation of an embryo. If the corpus luteum does not produce enough progesterone, then implantation may be difficult and the embryo may not survive. Also, if the corpus luteum starts to break down, and thus stops progesterone production before the embryo has implanted, implantation may also not occur.

Diagnosis

A blood test at seven days past ovulation (7 DPO) can confirm whether or not you have ovulated that cycle, by measuring the amount of progesterone your body has produced. The blood test can also tell if you are producing enough progesterone to sustain a pregnancy.

Another way to find out if you are ovulating every cycle and if your ovulation patterns are normal is to chart your fertility signs, in particular your waking temperature every morning. This is discussed in detail in Chapter 3.

Treatment

Some doctors will prescribe progesterone supplements for those who are ovulating but have low 7 DPO progesterone. These are usually taken from the day after ovulation. However, opinion is divided on whether this works or whether it is too late at this stage to make a difference. Another approach is to prescribe the drug Clomid to ensure a better quality of ovulation. Clomid is most commonly prescribed to those women who are not ovulating at all but it has also been shown to help women who do ovulate but have hormone imbalances that affect the quality of ovulation. However, because of the risk of multiple eggs, it is advisable to have an ultrasound before ovulation to make sure you aren't going to produce too many eggs.

Lifestyle issues

This is also, in effect, a hormonal problem. There are a number of lifestyle issues that can delay or prevent ovulation; this happens when these external stimuli have an impact on the hypothalamus and affect the production of the hormones that regulate the menstrual cycle. It is not uncommon for women to have a late ovulation or an anovulatory cycle once in a while.

Both physical and psychological stress can have an effect on the body and on ovulation. Illness, travel, exercise and rapid weight gain or loss can also have the same effect. However, all of these issues cause only a temporary change to the menstrual cycle; as soon as the cause of the change has ceased, your menstrual cycle should return to normal.

Alternative treatments

As with PCOS, acupuncture can help with hormonal imbalance in order to stimulate ovulation.

Support

www.irishinfertilitysupportforums.ie

Diminished Ovarian Reserve (DOR)

What does it mean?

Ovarian reserve refers to the quantity and quality of the eggs left in a woman's ovaries. Every woman is born with all the eggs that she will ever have; the number of eggs depletes as the woman ages. It is estimated that there are about two million eggs present at birth but only about four hundred thousand by the start of puberty. Each menstrual cycle sees hundreds of eggs start the journey to maturity, a journey that only one or two will complete. The eggs that do not make it to ovulation die and are reabsorbed into the ovary. The egg reserve continues to deplete throughout a woman's reproductive life, even while she is on the pill or pregnant.

Egg quality also diminishes over time. At puberty, only a small percentage of the eggs are of poor quality, but the good-quality eggs are the ones that are most likely to be recruited to ovulation. As time goes by, more and more of the good-quality eggs are used up and the percentage of poor-quality eggs increases. By the time a woman reaches her late thirties, she is likely to have a significantly larger proportion of poor-quality than good-quality eggs in her ovarian reserve. These poor-quality eggs are less likely to fertilise and more likely to miscarry if fertilisation does occur.

DOR usually refers to a marked decrease in the number of eggs available and the quality of those eggs. It is something that is expected in women over forty but can happen to women in their thirties and even in their twenties. It can also happen to women of any age as a result of cancer treatment. A diagnosis of DOR can come as a huge shock to those under forty, for whom infertility was previously not necessarily time-related; for some, it is the worst diagnosis they could have received. For those under forty, the condition is sometimes referred to as 'prematurely ageing ovaries'. Once FSH has risen to an extent that ovulation ceases completely, the condition is known as premature ovarian failure (POF).

Eggs are not replaceable, and there is no cure for prematurely ageing ovaries. For those with DOR, pregnancy is not impossible, although pregnancy rates are severely reduced, depending on the extent of the problem. For those who do conceive, miscarriage rates are very high, due to the high numbers of poor-quality eggs. The earlier DOR is diagnosed, the sooner fertility treatment can be organised; this problem is only likely to get worse over

How is it diagnosed?

There is no way of testing directly for DOR. An elevated level of follicle-stimulating hormone (FSH) early in the menstrual cycle has been strongly linked to a depleted egg reserve. At this stage of the cycle, the pituitary gland in the brain releases FSH to instruct the ovaries to start maturing the eggs in its follicles. The fewer eggs that are available for maturation, the more FSH is needed. So a high level of FSH at this stage is indicative of a DOR. Your FSH level can be measured by a blood test on day 2 or 3 of your cycle. It is important to measure oestradiol (E2) levels at the same time, as a seemingly normal FSH reading may be inaccurately low if the E2 level is abnormally high. FSH levels can vary from cycle to cycle but it is generally accepted that the highest level is the one that is indicative of ovarian reserve.

Levels below 10 are generally considered to be normal, although this should be cross-referenced with the woman's age, as women in their twenties and early thirties are usually expected to have FSH levels lower than 6. A woman in her twenties with an FSH level of 8 or 9 would be advised to seek further tests. It should also be noted that, while an FSH level above 10 is strongly linked to DOR, a level under 10 does not necessarily rule out the condition, especially if the woman is over thirty-five. Further testing may be required if no other cause of infertility has been found.

A further test for DOR is the Clomid challenge test (CCT). This is usually used to check the FSH levels of those who have had a normal result on their day-two or day-three test. FSH levels are tested on cycle day 10 after taking 100mg of Clomid from cycle days five to nine. The Clomid stimulates the pituitary to produce an excess of FSH, but if the ovary has a good reserve, then it will respond to the increase in FSH by producing more oestrogen, which will in turn feed back to the pituitary, thus reducing the FSH level. If FSH is below 10 on day 10, then a diminished reserve is unlikely. However, a poor reserve will usually return a high result on day 10, even if levels were normal on day 2 or 3.

An ultrasound to determine your antral follicle count (the number of follicles present in your ovaries at the start of your cycle, before they have begun to mature) can be performed on day 2 or 3 of your cycle. Four or more in each ovary usually suggests a normal ovarian reserve.

Another indicator of DOR is a poor response to FSH medication used to stimulate the ovaries in preparation for IVF. Usually, the higher the woman's FSH level, the fewer follicles are produced in response to stimulation, even at the highest doses of medication.

But – and it's a big but – although each of these tests is a good indicator of the quantity of eggs remaining, there is no easy way of measuring the quality of those eggs. It is usually assumed that a low quantity of eggs goes hand in hand with low quality, but this is not always the case, especially in women under forty. In fact, some doctors consider that chronological age is more closely related to egg quality, regardless of FSH level.

I am a good test case in this scenario. At the age of thirty-seven, my FSH was 17. On my first IVF, I produced only two good follicles, despite injecting the maximum dose of medication to stimulate my ovaries. Two eggs were collected, both were fertilised, and they produced good-quality embryos. I did become pregnant but miscarried soon afterwards. My doctor told me that as I produced eggs that 'wanted' to become embryos, I still had a good chance of becoming pregnant, despite my high FSH. He did not consider that my recurrent miscarriage problem was due to poor-quality eggs. However, the only way to assess egg quality is to undergo IVF and see the quality of embryos that are produced as a result.

What are the symptoms?

The early symptoms of DOR and rising FSH can be barely noticeable; this is the reason that a poor test result can come as such a shock. You may notice that your cycle has shortened, in particular the follicular phase. This is because an increase in FSH can cause the follicles to develop more quickly, and so you may ovulate earlier than before. You may also notice a shortened or irregular luteal phase, as a poor or varying quality of ovulation from cycle to cycle results in the corpus luteum degenerating before the 'normal' fourteen-day period. However, many women only begin charting their cycles when they have failed to conceive after a certain period of time. They may previously have been unaware of when they ovulated or how long their cycles were.

Again, I am not a typical high-FSHer when it comes to cycle length and follicular phase length in particular. I usually ovulate on or after CD14. I do have a short luteal phase – anything from seven to twelve days. However, my cycles have always been shorter than the average twenty-eight days and have always varied in length. Although I never kept track of my cycles before we started TTC, I never knew exactly what day my period would arrive – unlike most other women I know. So I don't know how, or even if, this is related to my high FSH.

As FSH rises to pre-menopausal levels, the symptoms include those associated with low oestrogen: hot flashes, night sweats and vaginal dryness.

However, these are not usually experienced by women with an FSH level between 10 and 20 who are still ovulating and still fertile to some extent.

How can it be treated?

There is no cure for DOR; eggs simply cannot be replaced. However, this does not mean that you cannot become pregnant. In fact, a quick read through *www.ivfconnections.com* or other message boards that deal with high FSH shows that many women who had been given little hope of having children went on to conceive naturally. Also, women who have had no problems having children have never had their FSH tested, so we just don't know how many women with high FSH are conceiving naturally and carrying to term. It can happen, but for many there is just no way of controlling how or when this may be.

However, high-FSHers, more than anyone, cannot afford to wait and see, as the problem is only likely to get worse over time. The treatment options are similar to those facing a diagnosis of unexplained infertility. Clomid can help to improve the quality of ovulation, ensuring your egg quality is as good as it can be. IUI with ovarian stimulation is also an option, but success rates are generally low.

By far the greatest success rates are seen in those women who undergo IVF. Although the number of eggs collected is usually well below average, if those eggs are of reasonable quality, the couple has some chance of pregnancy. There are certain IVF protocols that are more suited to women with high FSH, who are likely to have a poor response. There is a short protocol, which does not involve shutting down the ovaries prior to stimulation. Instead, ovarian stimulation medication begins on day 2 or 3 of the menstrual cycle and works in conjunction with the woman's own FSH. There is also a protocol that involves the woman taking oestrogen supplements prior to stimulation in order to try to improve her response to the stimulation with FSH medication. Often, you may have to try more than one protocol (and undergo more than one cycle of IVF) before you find the protocol that is best suited to your specific circumstances.

For those who do not produce any follicles during the IVF process, or those for whom eggs do not fertilise or embryos do not result in pregnancy, there is always the option of using donor eggs. It is estimated that 20 percent of IVF cycles use donated eggs; this can be a wonderful option for those who would not otherwise be able to achieve a pregnancy. There is more information on donor eggs in Chapter 7.

Alternative treatments

While Western medicine will tell you that there is no turning back the clock on high FSH – simply changing the amount of FSH used to stimulate your ovaries will not affect your ovarian reserve – many TCM practitioners disagree. While the number of eggs will continue to diminish, many practitioners believe that treatment with acupuncture and Chinese herbs, which can bring down FSH levels, can also result in a better quality of ovulation, leading to higher pregnancy rates.

Nina Liu of Melt in Temple Bar says that success rates depend on the person and that some have success with acupuncture alone, while others need an intensive course of herbs and acupuncture. Once the body and hormones are balanced and ovulation is occurring as normal, the woman has a much better chance of conceiving.

I have undergone acupuncture for the last two years, not because I had any evidence that it was doing me any good but simply because I wanted to ensure that I was doing everything possible to help me conceive. Last year I conceived naturally for the first time in two years. I can't put it down to any one aspect of my care – I had been looking after my diet, taking regular exercise, was on fertility drugs and was on pregnancy-support medication from ovulation – but it did happen at a time when my acupuncturist, Nina, felt that my body was in balance, and she told me beforehand that I had a good chance of conceiving during that cycle.

Support

www.irishinfertilitysupportforums.ie
www.ivfconnections.com
www.pofsupport.org

Uterine abnormalities

What are they?

Abnormalities of the uterus are a fairly uncommon cause of infertility. However, they are an important consideration during fertility investigations, and even if they are not found to be the cause of infertility, they may need to be treated, as some can have an adverse affect on pregnancy, resulting in premature labour or miscarriage. They can also be an important consideration when deciding on a course of fertility treatment. About 4.3 percent of women have a uterine abnormality, many without ever knowing it, as it has no effect on their fertility or on their ability to give birth.

Congenital uterine abnormalities

There are a number of congenital (developed before birth) uterine abnormalities, most of which have little effect on fertility. A bicornuate uterus is one that, instead of being pear-shaped, is shaped like a heart, with a deep indentation at the top. This means that the baby has less space to grow than in a pear-shaped uterus, and the pregnancy should be monitored closely because of the risk of preterm labour. A unicornuate uterus occurs when the uterine tissue does not develop properly, and is a very rare condition. A unicornuate uterus is half the size of a normal uterus, and the woman only has one fallopian tube but usually has two ovaries. This also requires careful monitoring, in case of premature labour. A double uterus is when the uterus has two inner cavities. Each may have its own cervix and vagina. Again, this is very rare. An arcuate uterus has a single uterine cavity with a convex or flat uterine fundus, the upper portion of the uterus, where pregnancy occurs. An arcuate uterus does not usually cause problems for fertility or pregnancy.

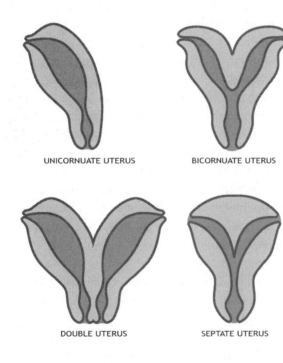

UNICORNUATE UTERUS   BICORNUATE UTERUS

DOUBLE UTERUS   SEPTATE UTERUS

Fig. 6.3 Congenital uterine abnormalities

A septate uterus is the most common form of congenital uterine abnormality and the most highly associated with infertility and miscarriage. In a septate uterus, the inside of the uterus is divided by a wall or septum. The septum may extend part of the way into the uterus or can reach as far as the cervix. It is estimated that one in four women with this condition will suffer from infertility. This is because the septum has no blood flow and can interfere with implantation. Treatment usually involves surgical removal of the septum either by hysteroscopy or laparoscopy (see page 114).

Some uterine abnormalities can be diagnosed with a simple ultrasound - a bicornuate uterus can often be seen clearly. However, even if a uterine abnormality can be identified using ultrasound, a hysteroscopy and/or a laparoscopy is usually used for a full diagnosis. Treatment can then be carried out also by hysteroscopy or laparoscopy either at the time of diagnosis or at a future date.

Acquired uterine abnormalities

In contrast to congenital uterine abnormalities that occur during foetal development, acquired uterine abnormalities develop after birth. The most common of these are intrauterine adhesions, endometrial polyps and uterine fibroids.

Intrauterine adhesions are made up of scar tissue that form in the uterus. In some cases, the scar tissue is so severe that the front and back walls of the uterus stick together; in other cases, adhesions occur only in small portions of the uterus. The most common cause is a dilation and curettage (D&C) after miscarriage, and they can also happen after an abortion, a caesarean section or uterine surgery. Symptoms include irregular or absent periods and pain during menstruation, although many women have no symptoms at all. The adhesions can prevent the sperm travelling to meet the egg and can also cause problems with implantation. Hysteroscopy is the most reliable method of diagnosis of intrauterine adhesions, and they can then be treated by laparoscopy (see page 114).

Endometrial polyps are small, benign growths of tissue on the lining of the uterus and are a frequent cause of abnormal uterine bleeding. Their role in infertility is not well understood, although they are thought to interfere with implantation. Approximately 3 to 5 percent of infertile women have endometrial polyps. They can be identified by ultrasound or by hysteroscopy. The majority of endometrial polyps can be removed by D&C, which involves dilating the cervix and scraping out the uterus. This is usually done under general anaesthetic.

Uterine fibroids are benign growths, made up of muscle cells and other tissues, that develop within the lining of the uterus. They are thought to affect up to 30 percent of women over thirty. They can grow on their own or in clusters and can vary in length from a few millimetres to about 20 centimetres. Symptoms include pain and heavy menstrual bleeding. Uterine fibroids can be subserosal (on the outside surface of the uterus), intramural (within the muscular wall of the uterus), submucosal (pushing into the uterine cavity) or pedunculated (attached by a stalk). The only type that is likely to have an impact on fertility (unless it is very large) is the submucosal type: because it pushes into the uterine cavity, it affects implantation and can also cause miscarriage. Uterine fibroids can usually be diagnosed by ultrasound, but a hysteroscopy or laparoscopy may also be needed (see page 114). The procedure to remove individual fibroids is known as myomectomy. (This procedure preserves fertility for women who wish to have children.). It can be done with the help of a hysteroscopy or a laparoscopy. Studies have shown that pregnancy rates after myomectomy in women with no other known fertility problems can be as high as 75 percent.

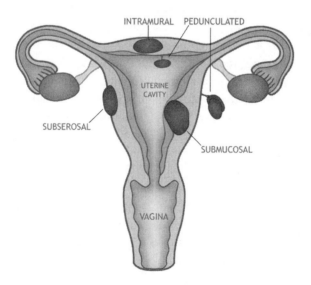

Fig. 6.4 Types of uterine fibroids

Diagnosis and treatment

Ultrasound, also known as sonography, is an imaging method that uses high-frequency sound waves to produce images of structures within the body. Pelvic ultrasound, which is used to view the uterus, can be conducted abdominally or transvaginally (through the vagina). An abdominal ultrasound involves putting a small handheld device (a transducer) on your abdomen. The transducer generates and receives high-frequency sound waves that cannot be heard by the human ear. The sound waves emitted by the transducer are reflected by the pelvis and transmitted to a computer, which generates images that can be viewed on a monitor. With a transvaginal ultrasound, the transducer is contained in a small rod, which is placed inside the vagina. Many women have a fear of transvaginal ultrasound but I can assure you that it does not hurt and is not usually even uncomfortable.

A hysteroscopy is a simple procedure that allows inspection of the uterus using a telescope-like instrument known as a hysteroscope. A local anaesthetic is usually injected around the cervix, and the uterus is inflated with carbon dioxide gas in order to give the doctor a better view of the uterus. The hysteroscope is then inserted into the vagina and through the cervix so that the uterine cavity can be examined. Images from the uterus are then displayed on a monitor. A hysteroscopy usually takes about thirty minutes.

A laparoscopy is a more complex procedure and usually involves a general anaesthetic. Firstly, the abdominal area is inflated with carbon dioxide gas so that the surgeon can see it properly. Then a small cut is made, usually in the navel, and the laparoscope (a microscope with a light on the end) is passed through it into the pelvic area. The images picked up by the laparoscope are displayed on a monitor. A laparoscopy is usually done as a day procedure.

Alternative treatments

There is little evidence that acupuncture or Chinese herbs alone can prevent or cure acquired uterine abnormalities, although some anecdotal evidence suggests that it can play a part. They can certainly help balance the body and the reproductive hormones in the aftermath of surgery.

Support

www.irishinfertilitysupportforums.ie

Blocked fallopian tubes

What does it mean?

Blockages in the fallopian tubes account for 20 to 25 percent of all female infertility. The fallopian tubes are the channels that connect the uterus to the ovaries; if these tubes are blocked, the sperm is unable to travel to meet the egg, and vice versa. Either one or both tubes may be blocked; problems can also arise when there is no tubal blockage but scarring or other damage on the fallopian tube.

Damage to the fallopian tubes is usually caused by pelvic infection, such as pelvic inflammatory disease (PID) or pelvic endometriosis. It can also be caused by scar tissue that forms after pelvic surgery. PID is an infection that can affect the uterus, ovaries, fallopian tubes and surrounding areas. It is usually caused by gonorrhea or chlamydia that travels from the cervix to the uterus and fallopian tubes. Symptoms include pain, heavy vaginal discharge and irregular or heavy periods. PID is usually diagnosed following a pelvic examination but a laparoscopy may be needed to confirm the diagnosis. It is usually treated successfully with antibiotics. Bacteria, white blood cells and other fluids fill the tubes as the body combats the infection. However, during the healing process, the delicate inner lining of the fallopian tubes can become permanently scarred and the end of the tube may become partially or completely blocked.

Another problem for those with tubal scarring or partial tubal blockage can be tubal ectopic pregnancy (see Chapter 9). This occurs when a fertilised egg implants in the fallopian tube instead of in the uterine lining: the blockage does not prevent the sperm from travelling to meet the egg but stops the fertilised egg from travelling to the uterus. Studies show that the rate of ectopic pregnancy in women who have had PID is six to ten times that of those who have no history of PID.

How is it diagnosed?

The first step towards diagnosing (or ruling out) blocked fallopian tubes involves an HSG (hysterosalpingogram). This is an x-ray examination, during which dye is injected through the cervix and into the uterine cavity. If the fallopian tubes are open, the dye flows through the tubes and spills out into the abdominal cavity. A series of X-rays are taken during this procedure in order to document the flow of the dye. The procedure takes about ten minutes and is not usually painful, although some women have reported varying degrees of pain when the cervix is opened in order to inject the dye. A couple of strong painkillers taken about half an hour before the procedure should be enough to ensure it is not too uncomfortable. You may also experience some cramping afterwards.

Even if the fallopian tubes are found to be open, this does not mean that the tubal function is normal. The inside lining of the tubes may contain scarring, and this can prevent a fertilised egg from travelling to the uterus. Hair-like cilia, which are located on the inside of the fallopian tubes, carry the fertilised egg to the uterus. A build-up of scar tissue can damage the cilia and prevent them from transporting the egg. This can result in either a lack of implantation or ectopic pregnancy. A laparoscopy (see page 114) can be performed to assess tubal damage that is not diagnosed by an HSG.

How can it be treated?

There are two options for women who suffer from damage to the fallopian tubes. The first is surgical repair of the fallopian tubes. The success of this surgery depends on the extent of the damage: not all blockages or scarring can be repaired. The surgery can usually be done by laparoscopy, although some may require a laparotomy, which requires a bigger incision in the abdomen.

The second option is for the couple to do IVF. This way, the egg (or eggs) is retrieved from the woman's ovary and is fertilised with the sperm in a laboratory; the resulting embryo is then transferred to the woman's uterus, thus bypassing the need for it to travel down the fallopian tube. The decision as to whether to opt for surgical repair of the tubes or IVF should be discussed extensively with your doctor and will be based on a number of factors: success rates, the existence of other infertility factors, the age of the woman and economic and other considerations.

Support

www.ivfconnections.com
www.irishinfertilitysupportforums.ie

Karen from Dundalk

I have had blocked fallopian tubes. It was first discovered when I had a HSG to find out why we weren't conceiving, and then I had a laparoscopy to confirm it. I was then referred to the Rotunda Hospital, where I had microsurgery to try to unblock the tubes. This isn't keyhole surgery. The reason it's called 'micro' is because the tools they use are extremely small in order to reduce further damage to the tubes. They used a laser to burn off any adhesions in my fallopian tubes. I was cut open in a similar way to a caesarean section and I had to spend five days in hospital.

My operation was technically a success because the tubes were free of adhesions and the dye could run through my tubes, but my doctor said he wouldn't fully know how successful it was until I got pregnant. I never did get pregnant on my own but I did manage to get pregnant with the help of IVF. There was no definite reason given for my adhesion but one doctor I attended thought it was from surgery I had had when I was eighteen.

Common medical conditions – for men

Poor sperm quality and quantity

What does it mean?

Men are just as likely to suffer from fertility problems as women: approximately 35 percent of cases of couples who have difficulty conceiving are as a result of male-factor infertility, with a further 20 percent of cases being a combination of male- and female-factor infertility. Male-factor infertility is usually indicated by a low quality or quantity of sperm present in a semen sample, and is therefore much easier to assess than female-factor infertility. A semen analysis, which measures the number and quality of sperm in a sample, along with some other factors, is one of the initial tests that should be conducted when a couple first present for infertility investigations. However, it is still common for medical practitioners to proceed with perhaps unnecessary tests and treatment for women without carrying out a simple semen analysis first. Obviously the discovery of a low quality or quantity of sperm does not rule out female-factor problems, but as soon as this problem is discovered, steps can be taken to improve the situation, thus giving the couple a better chance of achieving a pregnancy.

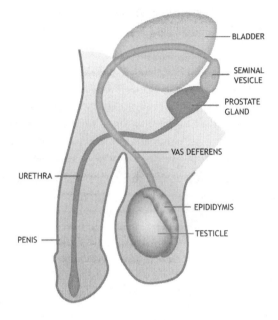

Fig. 6.5 The male reproductive system

Unlike women, who are born with all the eggs they will ever have, men produce sperm continuously, with each sperm cell taking about seventy-two days to reach maturity. The sperm are produced in the testes and are then stored for up to two weeks in the epididymis, where they mature, develop motility and become capable of fertilisation.

Problems with sperm can be caused by obstructions of the genital tract that block the flow of semen, thus resulting in an inadequate amount of semen being present in the ejaculate. These abnormalities can be congenital (present at birth) or can occur due to infection or surgery.

Another factor which should not be overlooked is of a psychosexual nature. Problems can arise from the defective delivery of sperm into the female genital tract, which can be caused by impotence or premature ejaculation. There are also several genetic disorders, such as cystic fibrosis, that can affect male fertility.

However, problems with the production and maturation of sperm are by far the most common causes of male infertility. Many things can interfere with the normal production and maturation of sperm, the most common ones being illness, medication, environmental and lifestyle factors, hormonal imbalances and varicoceles (varicose veins in the scrotum). The main problems that arise are with the number of sperm produced (count), the ability of the sperm to move properly (motility) and the shape and form of the sperm (morphology):

Sperm count

This is the number of sperm present per millilitre (ml) of semen in one ejaculation. A normal sperm count is considered to be greater than or equal to 20 million sperm per ml. Between 10 and 20 million is considered low, and anything below 10 million is very low. Sperm produced in very low numbers is known as oligospermia. Some men will have no sperm at all; this is known as azoospermia.

Sperm motility

This is a measure of the percentage of sperm that can move forward normally. This can often be of more importance than the sperm count. Motility is graded from A to D as follows:

Grade A (fast progressive) sperm are those that swim forward quickly and in a straight line.

Grade B (slow progressive) sperm swim forward but slowly or in a curved line.

Grade C (non-progressive) sperm move their tails but do not move forward.

Grade D (immotile) sperm do not move at all.

Fifty percent of the sperm need to be Grade A or B for the motility to be considered normal. Poor sperm motility is known as asthenospermia.

Sperm morphology

This is a measure of the percentage of sperm that have a normal shape. A good sperm should have an oval head with a connecting mid-piece and a long, straight tail. At least 15 percent of sperm should be normally shaped (as determined by the Kruger classification system – the WHO system, which is less rigid, expects 60 percent of sperm to be normally shaped) in order for the sample to be considered normal. Morphology of less than 15 percent is known as teratozoospermia.

A semen analysis will usually also consist of a test for anti-sperm antibodies. Some men produce antibodies to their own sperm that can impede the movement of sperm through the woman's cervical mucous, inhibit the binding of a sperm to the egg and inhibit the sperm's penetration into the egg. The semen should also be tested for the number of white blood cells: an unusually high number can be indicative of infection or inflammation.

Because sperm are constantly being produced, the count, motility and morphology can change on a regular basis. A follow-up semen analysis should be conducted about six weeks after the initial test.

What are the symptoms?

There are rarely any symptoms associated with poor sperm quality or quantity, unless it is caused by an infection or a physical blockage in the genital tract, in which case there may be some pain or discomfort. Generally, the only symptom of male-factor infertility is the inability to conceive after a year spent TTC.

What causes it?

There are a wide range of causes of poor sperm quality and quantity. Many, such as environmental and lifestyle factors, are transient, and the effects can be reversed as soon as the cause is stopped. These factors include smoking, the use of alcohol and recreational drugs, some medications, exposure to chemicals and toxins, excess weight, and the exposure of the testicles to high temperatures. The reason the testicles are located outside the body, in the scrotum, is that sperm production needs to take place slightly below normal body temperature. Therefore anything that increases the temperature of the testicles can cause an interference with sperm production and should be avoided. This includes hot baths, saunas, jacuzzis, prolonged sitting in one place, and any activity, such as long-distance cycling, that pushes the testicles back up towards the body.

In order to limit the effect of lifestyle and environmental damage to sperm quality and quantity, the following guidelines should be observed:

1. *Stop smoking*
   Studies show that this can dramatically reduce your sperm quality.

2. *Avoid recreational drugs*
   Marijuana can decrease sperm count, motility and morphology. Cocaine and opiates can contribute to erectile dysfunction, and amphetamines can decrease sex drive.

3. *Limit alcohol intake*
   Try to limit your alcohol consumption to three drinks, twice a week.

4. *Avoid saunas, jacuzzis and hot baths*
   Avoid all sources of excessive or prolonged heat, as these can affect sperm production and damage sperm quality.

5. *Take stretch breaks*
   Prolonged sitting at work, at home or in your car can increase your scrotal temperature and impair sperm production.

6. *Watch out for toxins*
   Be careful when handling workplace and household chemicals, as these may reduce sperm count and motility. Wear gloves and protective clothing where possible.

7. *Check all medications with your doctor*
   Many prescription medications can temporarily reduce your fertility.

8. *Ensure a healthy BMI (body mass index)*
   Men who are overweight have been shown to have lower sperm quality than those who have BMIs within the normal limits.

9. *Include essential vitamins in your diet*
   Vitamins C and E are powerful antioxidants that protect the sperm and contribute to increased concentration and better motility. Vitamin C is found in citrus fruits and Vitamin E is found in walnuts, almonds and vegetable oils such as sunflower and safflower. Zinc is also an essential mineral for the healthy formation and maturation of sperm. It can be found in pumpkin seeds, shellfish and red meat.

Other causes of poor sperm quality and quantity include physical abnormalities such as blockages of the genital tract and varicoceles, infections, immune-system disorders, hormonal abnormalities and genetic disorders.

How can it be treated?

In about 50 percent of men with poor sperm quality or quantity, the cause of the condition is treatable. These factors include varicoceles, ductal blockages, immune-system disorders, hormonal abnormalities and infections. A varicocele can raise the temperature of the scrotum, thus interfering with sperm production. It can be removed surgically; approximately 70 percent of those who undergo a varicocele ligation see an improvement in sperm quality, and in most cases that improvement is in sperm motility. Surgery can also help with blockages and scarring in the genital tract.

Immune-system disorders, whereby antisperm antibodies are produced, can be treated with steroids. Hormonal abnormalities can also be treated with medication. HCG (human chorionic gonadotrophin) can support the production of testosterone, and Clomid can help regulate LH (luteinising hormone) and FSH (follicle-stimulating hormone), which can in turn regulate testosterone production. Infections can usually be treated with antibiotics.

The two forms of ART (assisted-reproduction technologies) available for those with male-factor infertility are IUI (intrauterine insemination) and IVF (in-vitro fertilisation). With IUI, the man produces a semen sample, which is then treated (in a process known as 'washing') to ensure that only the best-quality sperm remain. This sperm is then injected directly into the uterus of the man's partner, thus bypassing the need for the sperm to swim through the cervix. This technique has an overall success rate of about 12 percent but is generally only successful in those couples with slight male-factor infertility.

IVF has the highest pregnancy rate, at about 25 percent per cycle. This is slightly higher when male-factor infertility is not too severe and there is no known female-factor infertility. Success rates also depend on the age of the female partner. If the male-factor infertility, in particular the sperm count, is especially bad, a technique called ICSI (intracytoplasmic sperm injection) can be used. In ICSI, a single sperm is injected into each egg. IUI, IVF and ICSI are discussed in more detail in Chapter 7.

It is important to remember that a semen analysis showing less-than-normal parameters does not usually mean that a natural pregnancy is impossible; in most cases, it just means that your chances are reduced each cycle. For example, a count of 15 million per ml or motility of 30 percent is generally regarded as *sub*-fertile rather than *in*fertile, and while fertility treatment will increase the likelihood of pregnancy, it may not be a necessity. There are always reports on message boards of couples conceiving while waiting for IVF due to male-factor infertility. It is really up to both of you to decide whether you are prepared to keep trying with reduced odds or to go straight for the treatment that will give you the best chance of achieving pregnancy.

Alternative treatments

Because sperm production depends on a number of factors, rebalancing the body using acupuncture has been shown to have a positive effect on sperm quality and quantity.

Nina Liu of Melt in Temple Bar claims that it is much easier to rebalance men's bodies than women's and that, therefore, improving male fertility is an easier job. She says that it depends on age and the severity of the problem but that most men should see an improvement in two to three months. She says that it is easier to improve motility than count and explains that most sperm problems are related to kidney deficiency and that most men suffer from this to a certain extent. Treating sperm problems therefore usually involves rebalancing the kidney. Men can also suffer from liver stagnation, which is easy to treat but involves cutting down on alcohol.

Support

www.irishinfertilitysupportforums.ie

John from Dublin

Before all the trouble started, we got pregnant on our first attempt, which wasn't even a particularly planned attempt. So we had private jokes about my super-sperm. It turns out it wasn't so super at all. It seems very odd now, looking back, that we were receiving fertility treatment for several months before some bright spark thought it'd be a good idea to get *me* checked out too. The sperm count was OK but sperm motility was bad, which means I had plenty of tadpoles but their swimming was as good as my walking after eight pints.

This didn't bother me: not in a male-pride kind of way, anyway – I'm not the macho type. But deep down I think I was glad that it was motility and not sperm count: a bloke's sperm motility is not something I've ever heard being called into question. So off I went to the 'ball doctor' and got on to the couch. He had a rummage around and straight away found that I had a varicocele, which is pretty much like varicose veins on your nads. I knew I'd developed some lumpy veins on one side since I was a teenager but didn't think it was anything to worry about. It was hardly noticeable. He explained that it was very common and didn't cause any harm but that it does increase the temperature in the area slightly, which can affect sperm quality. So I'd have to have it removed and the vein tied up. Ouch.

Well, the operation went fine. It was the most relaxing day I've had in years. I was sore for a few days after and couldn't run for a bus for weeks, but it was a success. We continued with fertility treatment, and after three IUIs and two IVFs we managed to conceive naturally. In the end, it was the varicocele ligation that won the day.

Unexplained infertility – for both partners

What does it mean?

Contrary to popular opinion, a diagnosis of unexplained infertility does not mean that there is nothing wrong with the couple. It certainly does not mean that going on a cruise, sharing a bottle of wine or just relaxing will help the couple become pregnant. A couple that has been diagnosed with unexplained infertility obviously suffers from infertility, yet both partners have undergone a diagnostic work-up that has failed to reveal the underlying cause of their infertility. It is a difficult diagnosis to come to terms with: on one hand, it can be a relief that no specific obstacle to becoming pregnant has been found; on the other, it can be difficult to accept that there are no obvious steps that can be taken to overcome the problems causing the infertility.

Unexplained infertility simply means that the cause of infertility has not yet been determined. Sometimes a couple may have basic tests (blood tests and a HSG for the woman; a semen analysis for the man) organised by their GP or gynaecologist, and an assessment of unexplained infertility may be made if the results of these tests are normal. Often the same couple, once they have been referred to a fertility clinic and have undergone more intensive testing, will find a specific reason for their infertility. So the diagnosis of unexplained infertility is not a definitive one and depends on the extent and accuracy of the infertility investigations that are conducted.

About 10 percent of infertile couples receive no explanation for their infertility after extensive investigations. A diagnosis of unexplained infertility does not mean that you can't or won't become pregnant. It does mean, however, that you will tend to have a substantially reduced fecundity rate – this is the chance of becoming pregnant in any given cycle. Couples with no fertility problems have approximately a 20 percent chance of conceiving each cycle; for those who have been diagnosed with unexplained infertility after a rigorous diagnostic process, the chances of becoming pregnant on any given cycle are somewhere between 1 and 4 percent.

How is it diagnosed?

For the male partner, a simple semen analysis (see previous section) is all that is needed to assess his fertility, although some doctors also recommend a post-coital test to check that the sperm move normally in the woman's cervical mucous. This test is usually done one to two days before ovulation, when the cervical mucous is thin, stretchy, plentiful and best suited for transporting sperm. The woman's cervical mucous is collected and examined within two to eight hours of the couple having sex. If you are tracking your fertility signs, you will have a good idea when you are coming up to ovulation. If not, then your doctor will probably advise you to keep an eye on your cervical mucous or use an ovulation-prediction test (which gives you between twelve and seventy-two hours' notice that ovulation is about to happen – see Chapter 2), or both.

For the female partner, a more in-depth analysis is needed. This involves a look at the woman's menstrual history, blood tests on day 3 of her cycle and at seven days past ovulation (7 DPO), and an HSG (hysterosalpingogram). The first thing a doctor will do is to try and establish that you are ovulating normally, thus ruling out PCOS and other ovulation problems. Your doctor will discuss your menstrual history to establish if your periods are regular and relatively pain-free. The next step is to have blood taken on day 2 or 3 of your cycle. This is to test the levels of hormones that regulate or affect your menstrual cycle (see Chapter 5). A further blood test at 7 DPO can check your progesterone levels to see if you have ovulated during that cycle.

If your hormone levels are normal and it has been established that you are ovulating, the next step is to check if your tubes are open. This is done by a procedure known as an HSG (see page 115). The results of the HSG may suggest that a laparoscopy (see page 114) is needed for further investigation.

If all these tests return as normal, a diagnosis of unexplained infertility is usually made. This does not mean that there is no reason for the couple's infertility; it simply means that no reason for the infertility has yet been found. Often the problem lies with egg quality, the ability of the sperm to fertilise the egg, and the ability of the embryo to implant in the uterine lining. All of these issues are difficult to assess.

How can it be treated?

Because there is no known problem causing the infertility, there is no one treatment path for couples who find themselves in this situation. There are a number of approaches and treatments that may work, however: the one you choose depends on how much you want to push yourselves physically, emotionally and financially.

Expectant management

This just means that you go home and keep trying every month in the hope that you will eventually conceive. The pregnancy rate for couples with unexplained infertility is somewhere between 30 and

60 percent at the end of three years of TTC. If you are not finding TTC too stressful and you are not yet ready to embark on a course of fertility treatment, this may be the option for you. However, many couples find the whole process of TTC so upsetting and stressful that the thought of having to wait until the end of three years for a slim chance of pregnancy is too much for them. Women in particular tend to want to be proactive in their treatment. As a result, most couples will not find this approach suitable.

Clomid

This is sometimes prescribed initially for those with unexplained infertility who want to do something but do not want to jump straight into more aggressive treatment. Clomid is an oestrogen-receptor modulator that acts on the pituitary gland to increase production of FSH (follicle-stimulating hormone) and LH (luteinising hormone). Clomid is usually prescribed for women who do not ovulate at all; the increase in hormones that it provides can stimulate the ovaries to develop and release an egg. In women who ovulate normally, the effect is usually to increase the quality and often quantity of eggs produced. This gives a better chance of fertilisation due to the better quality of ovulation and the chance that there may be two or more eggs available. Because of the risk of multiple pregnancy, an ultrasound prior to ovulation is advisable to determine how many follicles are growing in the ovaries.

The use of Clomid in cases of unexplained infertility is thought to increase the fecundity rate to about 5 percent. No increase has been reported after six cycles.

Intrauterine insemination (IUI)

IUI is a procedure in which a sample of sperm is deposited directly into the uterus, thereby bypassing the need for it to swim through the cervical mucous and navigate the cervix itself. A sample of semen is washed so that the best-quality sperm are available. Then a catheter is inserted through the cervix and into the uterus, and the washed sperm are injected through the catheter and into the uterus. IUI has been found to have a small benefit over timed intercourse in unexplained infertility, with fecundity rates rising to about 5 percent.

Success rates rise to about 10 percent when IUI is combined with ovarian stimulation. The woman's ovaries can be stimulated using Clomid or using gonadotrophins, such as Gonal-F or Puregon. Again, there is a risk of multiple ovulation, so ultrasound monitoring is usually advised.

In-vitro fertilisation (IVF)

IVF offers the highest pregnancy rate for those with unexplained infertility, with published figures ranging from 25 to 50 percent. It is high-tech, high-cost and high-stress, but many couples are prepared to bypass the other steps, opting for the treatment that offers the highest success rate.

The process of IVF involves the woman taking medication to shut down her menstrual cycle, then taking injections to stimulate her ovaries, in the hope that multiple eggs will be produced. Once these eggs have matured, they are retrieved from the ovaries by a fertility doctor; at this stage, the male partner is required to produce a semen sample. The sperm is then used to fertilise as many eggs as possible in a laboratory, and either two or three of any resulting embryos are transferred into the woman's uterus after three to five days. Any remaining embryos can then be frozen for use at another time.

Alternative treatments

TCM (traditional Chinese medicine, which involves acupuncture and herbs) looks at the functioning of the body as a whole, whereas Western medicine looks for problems with the component parts. TCM may observe an imbalance in the reproductive system when Western medicine has not found a specific reason for infertility. By improving the blood flow through the body, acupuncture and herbal treatment may stimulate a better quality of ovulation and help with implantation – both of which are problem areas that may not have been identified during the couple's diagnostic work-up. Anecdotal evidence suggests that long-term acupuncture treatment can aid pregnancy rates in women with unexplained infertility.

Reflexology has also been suggested as a method of promoting relaxation as well as blood and energy flow throughout the body. I could find no evidence linking it to an improvement in pregnancy rates, although anything that eases the stress associated with infertility has to be beneficial.

Support

www.irishinfertilitysupportforums.ie

7

Assisted-reproduction technologies

Introduction

Taking the first step on the path of fertility treatments can be a daunting prospect for many couples. For so long, you have thought that this next cycle might be the one to put an end to the misery and give you the two pink lines for which you've been waiting for so long. Every couple hopes to be one of those lucky couples that gets a positive test the week before the first appointment at the fertility clinic.

It may be scary, and it's certainly not the way you planned it, but by taking the assisted-reproduction route, you are giving yourselves the best possible chance of a pregnancy. It can be very expensive and stressful, however, so it is not something that should be embarked upon without careful consideration. However, I have to say that I found it less stressful than the never-ending process of unassisted TTC. Whether I was popping pills or sticking needles in my belly, I was focused, productive, and helping to give my body the best chance. It's not an easy time, especially if you have work or other commitments to keep, but if you have reached the stage where you and your doctors think you need treatment, it can often be a relief to get started on it.

The assisted-reproduction route doesn't always work. In fact, it might never work: that is the scariest part of the process. However, the more you learn about each treatment, the more you understand the range of options that are open to you. It is up to you how far you want to go, and how much you are prepared to endure.

Whether or not you decide to discuss your fertility journey with family and friends, it is unlikely that they will fully understand what you are going through unless they have been there themselves. Most couples, and in particular most women, find it very helpful to talk to others who are in the same boat. There are a number of options for those seeking support, and there are certainly plenty of other people out there who are going through the same trials and tribulations as you: one in six couples, to be precise. If you would like to talk to others face to face, you can contact the National Infertility Support and Information Group (NISIG), which holds bi-monthly support-group meetings throughout Ireland. NISIG is contactable by phone at 1890 647444 and 087 797 5058, by post at PO Box 131, Togher, Cork or by email at nisig@eircom.net. Their website is a *www.nisig.ie*.

For those who would prefer to meet others online, there is Ireland's first infertility-support forum, *www.irishinfertilitysupportforums.ie*, and also a busy TTC with Assistance board at *www.magicmum.com*, Ireland's busiest parenting site. For those undergoing IVF, *www.ivfconnections.com* has sections for all aspects of IVF, as well as local boards for your own country.

This chapter details the main fertility treatments that are available in Ireland. As yet, there is no legal framework governing the provision of assisted reproduction in Ireland (although guidelines have been laid down by the Irish Medical Council), and clinics vary in the services they provide. You should talk to your GP/gynaecologist and your local fertility clinics about the services they provide before you decide where to make an appointment.

Ovulation induction

Ovulation-induction medications, often referred to as fertility drugs, stimulate the ovaries to produce one or more mature follicles, in the hope that at least one egg will be released, which may then be fertilised. Ovulation induction on its own is not usually considered to be an assisted-reproduction technology (ART) because, once the egg has been released, the couple are left to their own devices to try to fertilise it. However, ovulation induction is usually used during the ART procedures IUI and IVF.

Who might benefit?

Ovulation induction without ART is usually indicated for those women who don't ovulate on their own, have irregular patterns of ovulation, or have hormonal imbalances in their menstrual cycles. It is also sometimes suggested as a first step for those suffering from unexplained infertility.

Ovulation induction can also be used to stimulate the ovaries and control the timing of ovulation for IUI and IVF. This is usually done using injectable gonadotropins; careful ultrasound monitoring is essential to avoid the risk of OHSS (ovarian hyperstimulation syndrome) and to monitor the number of follicles being produced.

What is the cost?

Thanks to the Drug Payment Scheme (see *www.citizensinformation.ie*), the cost of medication is never greater than €90 per month for an individual or a family.

There are three types of medication that are commonly used to induce ovulation: Clomid, Metformin and injectable gonadotropins. The drug HCG (human chorionic gonadotropin) is also often used to stimulate the release of the egg from the follicle.

Clomid (clomiphene citrate)

Clomid (the brand name of the drug clomiphene citrate) is the first port of call for many women who are looking for help to have a baby. It is cheap, easily available and prescribed by many GPs and gynaecologists, often without a full fertility work-up. This may be because it has been shown to give a slight increase in pregnancy rates for those suffering from unexplained fertility. However, it is advisable to get some basic tests done (as detailed in Chapter 5) before you embark on any course of treatment. Or you may, like me, find out after two months of taking Clomid that your partner has sperm problems and that it was all a waste of time and energy!

Clomid is an oral tablet that is usually taken each day for five days at the start of the menstrual cycle. It can be taken as early as days two to six or as late as days five to nine. Dosages start from 50mg a day. If there is no improvement in ovulation over two to three cycles, your doctor may increase the dose to 100mg or even 150mg.

Clomid works by tricking the body into believing that its oestrogen levels are low. As a result, the hypothalamus in the brain begins to secrete increased levels of GnRH (gonadotropin-releasing hormone), which in turn causes the pituitary gland, also in the brain, to release more FSH (follicle-stimulating hormone) and LH (luteinising hormone). The increase in the levels of these hormones should stimulate the ovaries to release one or more eggs. (There is more on how these hormones work in Chapter 2.)

Side effects

Different people have different reactions to Clomid: some, like me, have no side effects at all, while others suffer from mood swings, hot flashes and breast tenderness. Clomid may also cause less cervical mucous than usual to be produced and can result in a thinner than usual uterine lining. Because of the chance of multiple follicles, you may also have some discomfort in your ovaries in the days before ovulation, as they may swell to a greater than usual size.

Some doctors are happy to prescribe Clomid without follicle tracking, i.e. ultrasound monitoring of your follicles in the run-up to ovulation. Ideally, it should be done as a rule because of the risk of multiples. Approximately 10 percent of Clomid pregnancies are multiple pregnancies. Now, most infertiles will confess that that is the dream – two for the price of one! – but the reality is that multiple pregnancies are more risky for both mother and baby and have higher miscarriage and preterm-delivery rates. And while you might relish the idea of twins, what about sextuplets? This happened to one lucky couple last year after taking Clomid! Most clinics are happy to let couples proceed with a maximum of three to four follicles. Monitoring will also allow your doctor to see if you are indeed ovulating, and how well you are responding to the prescribed dose of Clomid.

Another thing to look out for is that Clomid can cause an OPK (ovulation prediction kit – see Chapter 2) to turn positive before an LH surge, so bear this in mind if you are using OPKs in the two to three days following your last pill.

Success rates

Clomid has good success rates for those suffering from anovulation. Fifty to eighty percent will start to ovulate, and for those with no other fertility problems, pregnancy rates are comparable to those of the general population. Overall, pregnancy rates for those who ovulate are reported to be about 50 percent over six cycles, with most pregnancies occurring in the first three to four months. It is not recommended that Clomid be prescribed for more than six months: it has been shown not to increase pregnancy rates after that length of time, and some research suggests that long-term use may increase the risk of ovarian cancer.

Clomiphene citrate is also available under the brand name Serophene in the US.

Glucophage (metformin)

Metformin (brand name Glucophage) is not in itself an ovulation-induction drug but it can help those with PCOS (polycystic ovarian syndrome – see Chapter 6) to ovulate by helping to regulate hormones. Metformin has previously been used to help control blood-glucose levels in those with Type 2 diabetes.

The drug works by decreasing the absorption of carbohydrates through the intestines, reducing the production of glucose by the liver, and increasing the sensitivity of muscle cells to insulin – the hormone that delivers glucose to the cells, where it is burned as fuel or stored. Women with PCOS frequently have insulin resistance, a condition where excessive amounts of insulin are required to transport glucose to cells. These high levels of insulin cause an overproduction of androgens (male hormones); this can interfere with the hormones that regulate menstruation and can result in a lack of ovulation. Metformin helps the body to transport glucose with less insulin, thus reducing both insulin levels and androgen production. With androgens at normal levels, the hormones of the menstrual cycle should return to the levels at which they can stimulate ovulation to occur. Metformin can also assist with weight loss, which can help balance menstrual hormones and stimulate ovulation. The usual dose of Metformin is 850mg twice daily, with 850mg three times daily considered the maximum safe dose.

Side effects

The most common side effects of taking metformin are nausea, vomiting, gas, bloating, diarrhoea and loss of appetite. These symptoms occur in about 25 percent of patients and may be severe enough for treatment to be stopped in about 5 percent of patients. The side effects are related to the dosage and may decrease if the dosage is reduced.

Success rates

The use of metformin for ovulation induction is relatively new; it is generally used once Clomid alone has not been effective. Trials have found, however, that the use of Clomid and metformin together is more effective in stimulating ovulation in those with PCOS than Clomid alone. Some research also suggests that metformin may reduce the risk of miscarriage and the incidence of gestational diabetes among PCOS sufferers. Because metformin reduces androgen production, it can also help reduce the other symptoms of PCOS, such as hair loss and increased body and facial hair, and aid weight loss. It is usually effective after two to three months' use.

Injectable gonadotropins

Gonadotropins are so called because they stimulate the gonads – the testes in men and the ovaries in women. Unlike Clomid, which works to stimulate the pituitary to increase FSH and LH production, these gonadotropins work directly on the ovaries in an attempt to stimulate follicle development. They are usually prescribed for ovulation induction in conjunction with IUI and

IVF but are also used for those for whom Clomid has not resulted in ovulation.

These medications are given by intramuscular (into muscle) injections or subcutaneous (under the skin) injections on a daily basis. The injections are started early in the menstrual cycle and are continued for approximately eight to fourteen days until one or more mature follicles are seen with ultrasound examination of the ovaries. At that point, an injection of HCG (human chorionic gonadotropin) is usually given to induce ovulation to occur approximately thirty-six hours later.

A variety of medications fall into the category of gonadotropins, with recombinant FSH (follicle-stimulating hormone) and HMG (human menopausal gonadotropin) being the main ones used for ovulation induction. GnRH (gonadotropin-releasing hormone) can also be used. HCG is used to induce ovulation rather than to stimulate follicle growth.

Recombinant FSH (Gonal-F, Puregon – also known as Follistim)

This form of FSH, known as follitropin, is produced synthetically but is identical to naturally occurring FSH. It is injected subcutaneously (under the skin) and stimulates the ovaries directly to mature follicles in preparation for ovulation.

The amount of FSH that is injected usually has a direct effect on the number of follicles that are produced. So for simple ovulation induction, a small dose (37.5 to 75iu) is used, unless there is evidence that more stimulation will be needed to mature a follicle. For IUI, one or two follicles is usually ideal, so 75 to 150iu of FSH is generally prescribed. Higher doses (from 150 to 600iu) are needed for IVF, as the greater the number of follicles produced, the more eggs are collected and the greater the chance of a healthy embryo being produced that will result in pregnancy. Very careful monitoring by ultrasound is essential at these higher doses of FSH, as there can be a risk of OHSS (ovarian hyperstimulation syndrome – see page 135).

Many couples are uncomfortable with the idea of injectables, as it seems such a big step up from popping a pill. When it comes to injectable FSH, the manufacturers have made it as simple as possible. There are no syringes, just a 'pen' into which a cartridge of FSH is loaded, with a small needle at the nib of the pen. As these injections are subcutaneous, the easiest place to inject is into the fatty area of the tummy, about an inch either side of, or below, the belly button. Swab down the area with an alcohol wipe first, grab an inch or so of flab, and push the pen into the skin at a 90 degree angle. It may sting a little but it shouldn't hurt much. Push the base of the pen in slowly and then wait for about ten seconds before removing it. Push down on the area for about twenty seconds afterwards to minimise bruising.

HMG (Menopur)

HMG is a purified extract taken from the urine of postmenopausal women. It contains both FSH and LH. It can be injected subcutaneously or intramuscularly.

Menopur is prescribed in vials of 75iu of powder, which must be mixed with diluents before injecting. The number of vials prescribed will depend on the treatment you are having (simple ovulation induction, IUI or IVF) and how much stimulation your ovaries are likely to need: the greater the number of vials used, the more your ovaries will be stimulated. As with FSH injections, ultrasound monitoring is essential to minimise the risk of OHSS (see page 135) and to monitor your follicle development.

The use of Menopur is slightly more complicated than Gonal-F or Puregon, as you need to mix the powder and diluent first. The diluent is drawn up into a syringe via a large needle and injected into the powder; the solution is then drawn back up into the syringe. A new needle can then be placed on the syringe in preparation for your injection. A subcutaneous injection needs a smaller needle than an intramuscular one. Before you inject, point the needle upwards, tap the syringe to force any air bubbles to the top, and then depress the plunger to force the air out. Swap down the area (tummy for subcutaneous, thigh or bum for intramuscular) with an alcohol wipe, grab an inch of flab, and push the needle into the skin at a 90 degree angle. Subcutaneous injections may sting a little but shouldn't hurt much. Intramuscular injections can be a little more painful, and the area can be numbed first (with Ametop gel) if necessary. Push the plunger in slowly, then wait for about ten seconds before removing it. Push down on the area for about twenty seconds afterwards to minimise bruising.

Side effects

Some common side effects of gonadotropin injections can be soreness or redness at the injection site, lower-abdominal tenderness, fluid retention, headaches, fatigue, breast soreness and mood swings. After a few days, you may get some pain or a feeling of 'fullness' in your ovaries, as you may be maturing more follicles than usual. If you experience any breathlessness, dizziness or nausea, or abdominal pain that is more than just discomfort, call your doctor immediately to ensure that you are not at risk of developing OHSS.

OHSS (ovarian hyperstimulation syndrome)

OHSS is a serious condition that happens as a result of over-stimulation of the ovaries. It is usually only a risk at higher levels of stimulation (such as those used for IVF); it affects approximately 1 percent of those patients. OHSS occurs when too many follicles develop, the ovaries become enlarged, and fluid seeps into the abdominal cavity. While many women using fertility drugs report discomfort during the time of ovulation, those who experience OHSS report severe abdominal pain and discomfort, breathlessness, nausea and a decrease in the amount of urine passed.

It is not known exactly what causes OHSS, although certain patients are considered more at risk than others. Women who are under thirty, who are underweight, who have PCOS, who have had a previous occurrence of OHSS, or who produce a large number of eggs or follicles and have high oestrogen levels are at a higher risk of developing OHSS.

The best way to prevent OHSS is by careful ultrasound monitoring during stimulation injections. Your doctor may also wish to do blood tests to check your oestrogen levels. You should also be vigilant and report any symptoms you think may be related to the injections. If your doctor suspects OHSS, it may be recommended that you stop stimulating your ovaries. You may be allowed to 'coast' for several days, whereby your follicles are allowed to develop without stimulation. During this time, you should have frequent blood tests to assess your response. All going well, you should then be allowed to proceed with treatment as planned. If you are doing IVF, there is another option: your doctor may opt to collect your eggs, fertilise them and then freeze any resulting embryos for transfer at a later date, when you have recovered from your OHSS symptoms.

Although OHSS can become severe and can even result in death, this is very rare. There has been one tragic death from OHSS in Ireland. A 2007 report found problems with the management of this particular patient's hospital care, and new recommendations were made for the management of OHSS in Ireland.

Success rates

Between 70 and 90 percent of anovulatory women can have ovulation induced with injectable gonadotropins. Pregnancy rates are better than with Clomid, and success rates of up to 15 percent per cycle can be achieved when combined with IUI – and about 30 percent with IVF. Success rates using recombinant FSH have been found to be similar to those using HMG.

Some research suggests that the use of HMG may result in fewer intermediate-sized follicles, which may reduce the risk of OHSS.

GnRH

GnRH works on the pituitary gland to stimulate the release of FSH and LH from the ovaries. It is often used in conjunction with other gonadotropins to control ovulation and to prevent a spontaneous LH surge: in this way, ovulation can be delayed until one or more follicles have reached maturity. GnRH can be administered by injection (Orgalutran) or in the form of a nasal spray (Suprecur).

A GnRH pump can also be used to induce ovulation. The pump must be worn all the time and is connected subcutaneously by a needle. It releases a small amount of medication into the body every sixty to ninety minutes. This form of treatment is more effective for women with hypothalamic amenorrhea, which is a relatively rare condition. It is less effective for inducing ovulation in women with other types of anovulation.

HCG (Pregnyl, Ovidrel)

This drug, derived from the purified urine of pregnant women, is generally used for triggering ovulation and is administered subcutaneously. Ovulation usually occurs about thirty-six hours after the injection. This is extremely useful for timing sexual intercourse, IUI and egg collection for IVF. It can also be used during the luteal phase of the menstrual cycle (post-ovulation) to help sustain the corpus luteum so that progesterone production is maintained and the uterine lining continues to build.

HCG is the hormone that is produced during pregnancy by the embryo as soon as it implants in the uterine lining. It is also the hormone that is measured by pregnancy tests, so the HCG from your injection will indeed turn a pregnancy test positive. In order to see if you are actually pregnant (i.e. your positive pregnancy test is as a result of an implanted embryo and not leftover HCG from your shot), you will need to give the shot time to leave your system. The length of time that the HCG stays in a person's system depends on the amount administered and the metabolism of the individual. For timed sexual intercourse and IUI, the dose is usually 5,000iu, whereas for IVF, 10,000iu is more commonly used. A rule of thumb is that half of the HCG leaves the system every twenty-four hours. Thus, a shot of 5,000iu HCG would decrease as follows:

Day 1	5,000
Day 2	2,500
Day 3, ovulation day	1,250
Day 4, 1 DPO	625
Day 5, 2 DPO	313
Day 6, 3 DPO	156
Day 7, 4 DPO	73
Day 8, 5 DPO	37
Day 9, 6 DPO	18
Day 10, 7 DPO	9
Day 11, 8 DPO	5
Day 12, 9 DPO	Trigger gone

The body has about 5iu HCG when not pregnant, so anything above that level is considered positive for pregnancy. The average HPT measures a level of 20 to 50iu HCG, so a positive test after about 8 DPO should not be a false positive. Be warned, though, pregnancy-test strips bought over the Internet can catch about 10iu HCG: I know this because I was getting very faint lines when my HCG blood level (beta) was 10.

HCG injections need to be prepared in much the same way as Menopur does. Each box of 5,000iu contains a vial of diluent and a vial of power. The diluent is drawn up into a syringe via a large needle and injected into the powder; the solution is then drawn back up into the syringe. If you are using 10,000iu, you can inject the solution in the syringe into another vial of powder and draw the resulting solution back into the syringe. A new needle can then be placed on the syringe in preparation for your injection. The injection is administered subcutaneously, so the best place is in the fat of your tummy, about an inch either side of, or below, your belly button. Before you inject, point the needle upwards, tap the syringe to force any air bubbles to the top, and then depress the plunger to force the air out. Swab down the tummy area with an alcohol wipe, grab an inch of flab, and push the needle into the skin at a 90 degree angle. Leave the needle in for ten seconds before withdrawing it and then push down on the area for about twenty seconds afterwards to minimise bruising.

Side effects

Many women experience no side effects at all, while others report symptoms that are typical of early pregnancy, such as tiredness, breast tenderness, bloating and mood swings. There may also be some redness or irritation at the injection site.

IUI: Intrauterine Insemination

IUI involves the injection of a sample of prepared sperm into the woman's uterus at the time of ovulation. The aim is to transport the best-quality sperm that is available as close to the egg as possible in the hope that it will give a better chance of pregnancy than intercourse. It is a low-tech form of ART and is much easier on the woman's body, less intrusive and less expensive than IVF.

Who might benefit?

IUI is most successful in cases of mild male-factor infertility, especially when motility is below average. As they are placed as close to the egg as possible, the sperm have less distance to swim and a greater chance of reaching the egg. It is also useful for those women who have poor or little cervical mucous – which is usually needed as a medium in which the sperm can swim up the cervix and into the uterus. As the sperm is placed directly into the uterus, there is no need for good-quality mucous in the cervix. IUI is also often prescribed as a preliminary treatment for unexplained infertility.

What is the cost?

IUI is not provided by the public-health service in Ireland, and the cost of having the treatment done privately ranges from about €500 to about €700 per cycle, depending on the clinic and the treatment protocol. Unfortunately, none of this is covered by any health-insurance providers. The HARI unit at the Rotunda in Dublin does run a public clinic, but the waiting list is very long. The Merrion Fertility Clinic in Dublin and the Galway Fertility Unit at the University Hospital offer a discount to patients who hold medical cards. Thanks to the Drug Payment Scheme (see *www.citizensinformation.ie*), the cost of medication is never greater than €90 per month for an individual or a family.

How does it work?

An IUI can be 'natural' (i.e. without the use of ovarian stimulation) or 'medicated' (i.e. combined with stimulation), either with Clomid or, more commonly, with injectable gonadotropins, administered in small doses. Even if you do not have ovulation problems, stimulation will provide you with a greater chance of more follicles being produced, giving a higher chance of pregnancy. It also makes the timing of ovulation easier to control. Ultrasound monitoring is essential whether stimulation is used or not, in order to determine when the follicle (or follicles) is mature and ready for

ASSISTED-REPRODUCTION TECHNOLOGIES

ovulation. This is usually when the dominant follicle (or follicles) reaches a size of 16 to 18mm. At this stage, a shot of HCG is generally administered to stimulate the ovary to release the egg or eggs. Ovulation will occur approximately thirty-six hours later; this is the time when the IUI should take place. Your clinic will organise the timing of your IUI and advise you when to take your HCG shot. IUIs tend to take place in the morning, so you can give yourself the HCG shot two nights previously. However, I did have one IUI that was scheduled for 4 PM, the only time they could fit me in. I had to get up at 4 AM the previous morning to take my HCG shot!

A couple of hours before the IUI is scheduled to take place, the male partner gives a semen sample at the clinic. This is then 'washed' so that only the best-quality (most motile) sperm are used in the IUI. The procedure itself involves a fine catheter being inserted through the cervix and into the uterine cavity; the sperm are then injected through this and into the uterus. IUI is generally painless (although you may feel a little bit of cramping afterwards) and only takes about fifteen minutes. You will probably be left to lie still and relax for a while afterwards, although there is no chance that the sperm will leak out if you do not rest.

IUI with donor sperm

In cases of severe male-factor infertility, couples may decide to use sperm from a donor. If successive semen analyses show the male partner to be azoospermic (a complete absence of sperm in the semen), or if other fertility treatments have failed, the couple may choose to use donor sperm. This is a very personal decision and one that is not arrived at lightly, with counselling being advocated by all clinics, but it can be a wonderful way in which a couple can have a baby. There is more information on donor sperm on page 157.

What are the success rates?

IUI success rates range from about 8 to 18 percent per cycle and depend on many factors: the type of infertility, whether or not ovarian stimulation has been used, the age of the woman, and the quality of sperm used. The greatest success rates are seen in couples with mild male-factor infertility, especially when the motility is below average but not severely reduced, i.e. between 25 and 50 percent motile sperm.

Patricia from Dublin

When my husband's semen analysis showed only 26 percent motility, we braced ourselves for fertility treatment. When the second sample was slightly worse than the first, we decided to do IUI. It wasn't that simple. Our clinic said we should wait for six months, as there was still a chance we could conceive on our own. We were devastated, as we had already been trying for two years. But what could we do? So we waited and waited, and kept trying on our own – to no avail. So when our next appointment came round six months later, we were ready for IUI. Then we were told I would have to have an HSG to check that my tubes weren't blocked. We were very disappointed that we hadn't been advised to have this done during the six-month wait. So we waited another couple of months, did the HSG, and got the all-clear. Finally, we could start IUI. Nope. We had to have regulatory blood tests. Be warned: there are certain blood tests that all couples undergoing fertility treatment must have. Make sure you get these done in plenty of time before your treatment starts, or it might be delayed.

By the time we'd had our blood tests, we were so wound up that we were just waiting for something else to go wrong. Thankfully, it didn't. Because I was ovulating on my own, we were to have a natural IUI: no stimulation injections, just an HCG injection to trigger ovulation when my follicle got big enough. The IUI itself was virtually painless – much like having a cervical smear. The two-week wait was agony, and I caved in on day 10 and did a test. Positive! My only regret is that we didn't insist on doing the IUI about eight months earlier.

IVF: In Vitro Fertilisation

IVF refers to the process whereby a woman's eggs are fertilised outside her body (literally, 'in glass'), and any resulting embryos are then transferred back into the uterus two to five days later. An IVF cycle involves many steps and can take from six to eight weeks. It can be a very stressful time, both physically and emotionally, as there are hurdles that must be overcome at each stage of the process. However, you may also feel a certain amount of relief that you have finally started on the process that will give you the best possible chance of pregnancy.

Who might benefit?

IVF is often viewed as a last-resort treatment, and many clinics will only advise it when other treatments (ovulation induction, IUI) have failed. However, there are many couples for whom any other treatment is likely to be a waste of time and who should be advised to proceed straight to IVF. That includes those with blocked fallopian tubes, some of those with endometriosis, and those with severe male-factor infertility. Also, women with high FSH levels should be advised to try a carefully tailored IVF protocol, as other treatments have a low chance of success. For those who have reached the stage of premature ovarian failure, IVF with donor eggs is likely to offer the only chance of pregnancy.

There is also the issue of the emotional toll that dealing with infertility can take on a couple. A couple that presents at a fertility clinic after three years of TTC may already be at the end of their tether and may be daunted by the prospect of spending six months on Clomid followed by another six months of IUI – with relatively low odds of success at the end of the process. Most couples agree that TTC gets progressively harder over time. In general, couples prefer to try low-tech, low-cost options first, but some consideration should be given to those couples who, when presented with all the facts, feel willing and able to proceed to IVF before all other options have been exhausted.

What is the cost?

The cost of IVF in Ireland ranges from €3,500 to €4,500 for a fresh cycle. Assisted hatching costs about €500, blastocyst transfer about €1,000, and ICSI about €1,000. Donor sperm costs an extra €400 or so, while a cycle of IVF with donor eggs costs about €8,000 in total. A frozen-embryo transfer costs approximately €1,200 per cycle.

IVF is not available on the public-health system in Ireland, nor is it covered by any of the private health insurers. The HARI unit at the Rotunda in Dublin does fund a small number of public patients, and the Merrion Fertility Clinic in Dublin and the Galway Fertility Unit at the University Hospital offer a discount to patients who hold medical cards. The Cork Fertility Centre offers IVF to medical-card patients under certain circumstances, but each case is decided on a discretionary basis.

Thanks to the Drug Payment Scheme (see *www.citizensinformation.ie*), the cost of medication is never greater than €90 per month for an individual or a family.

What does it involve?

There are a number of different protocols for IVF; the one your doctor chooses for you will depend on your infertility history and your age. Some protocols involve an initial period of downregulation (see below), while others begin at the stimulation stage. Often, especially with unexplained infertility, a first IVF can be as much a diagnostic as a treatment tool, as in this cycle, a great deal of new information can be acquired about a woman's ovarian response and egg quality. If a subsequent fresh cycle is needed, it can then be tailored more accurately to the specific needs of the couple.

1. *Downregulation*

   Most IVF protocols contain a period of downregulation, during which the ovaries are shut down or suppressed so that they do not produce follicles of their own accord. The first phase of this usually involves taking the birth-control pill (BCP) for a minimum period of two to three weeks. Most clinics will schedule your dates for egg collection and embryo transfer in advance, and the amount of time you spend on BCPs will depend on when you are booked in for those procedures.

   The second phase of downregulation involves the use of GnRH (gonadotropin-releasing hormone), which is usually administered via a nasal spray or by injection. This is administered for two to three weeks, after which you will have a transvaginal ultrasound to check that you have downregulated satisfactorily. You should expect to see no follicles in your ovaries and your endometrial lining should be thin.

2. *Ovarian stimulation*

   Once the hormones of your menstrual cycle have been suppressed, you have control over the stimulation of your ovaries. This is usually done with injectable gonadotrophins (FSH or HMG – see the section on ovulation induction), which are administered daily for a period of about seven to fourteen days, depending on your response. During this time, you will have regular transvaginal ultrasounds in order to determine how your ovaries are responding to the medication and how many follicles they are producing. You may also have blood tests to check your hormone levels. Your medication can be altered during this time if your doctor feels that you are not producing enough follicles or are in danger of producing too many.

Once enough follicles have developed to a suitable size (usually 16 to 22mm), a shot of HCG is taken in order to trigger ovulation; this occurs approximately thirty-six hours later. This shot is usually administered at night at home, with a view to having egg collection two mornings later.

3. *Egg collection*

Egg collection is carried out under local anaesthetic. However, the sedative used can have different effects on different women: some report feeling woozy, while others (including me) are knocked out for a couple of hours. Either way, you will probably not feel or be aware of much during the procedure. During this procedure, the ovaries are monitored by transvaginal ultrasound and a long, thin needle attached to the ultrasound probe is passed through the vaginal wall and into the follicles. The fluid in each follicle is aspirated (gently sucked out into the needle) and then examined for the presence of an egg. While you are in theatre, your partner will produce a semen sample, which can then be prepared immediately. When you come round, your doctor will probably let you know how many eggs have been collected. Approximately 70 to 80 percent of follicles contain eggs.

4. *Fertilisation*

As soon as the eggs are retrieved, they are sent to the embryologist, who will prepare them to undergo fertilisation. The embryologist will call you, usually the following day, to give you the 'fertilisation report', which lets you know how many eggs have fertilised and how they are doing. The average fertilisation rate is about 66 percent. The wait for this report is probably the worst part of IVF for the couple.

Fertilisation should be completed by the end of the first day after egg collection. By day 2, cell division should have begun. About 90 percent of fertilised eggs should divide every twelve to twenty-four hours after fertilisation, and they should have between two and four cells by day 2. Sometimes during cell division, fragmentation of the cells may occur. If this is significant, it may indicate that the embryo is dying. If there are only one to three good embryos on day 2, transfer can take place on that day. By day 3, embryos should have four to eight cells. If your doctor advises that transfer should be on day 3 and there are more than two to three good embryos available, the remaining embryos can be frozen for use at a future date.

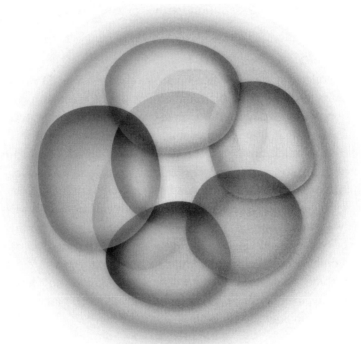

Fig. 7.1 Eight-cell embryo

Your doctor may suggest that the embryologist performs 'assisted hatching' on your embryos. This is where part of the outer shell of the embryo is scratched off to give the embryo a better chance of implanting in the uterine lining. This is advised for women over the age of thirty-seven, for those with high FSH, and for poor-quality embryos or those with a thick outer shell. Assisted hatching is performed shortly before embryo transfer.

5. *Embryo transfer*

This usually takes place two to three days after egg collection, unless you have been advised that the embryos should be allowed to grow to blastocyst stage (see below). The best one to three embryos are selected for transfer, and any remaining good embryos can be frozen. Two are usually selected (if available) if the woman is under forty, and three may be transferred if she is over forty.

Embryo transfer does not usually require an anaesthetic. It is a simple theatre procedure that only takes a few minutes. It does, however, require a full bladder in order to ensure that the uterus is fully visible on the ultrasound monitor. The embryo transfer itself is usually painless, but the full bladder can be a source of discomfort. You will probably be advised to drink one and a half to two litres of water before you arrive at the clinic, and you may end up sitting in the waiting room in pain for some time. The trick is not to fill your bladder completely until ten minutes or so before you are due in theatre. So save half of that water until then.

During the procedure itself, a fine catheter is inserted through the cervix and into the uterine cavity. The embryos are loaded into the catheter and are transferred (squirted out of the catheter) into the uterus. You may see a flash on the screen as this happens. This flash is the embryos, air and carrier fluid passing out of the catheter into your uterus. The presence of the flash indicates a slightly higher chance of pregnancy.

Progesterone supplements, in the form of pessaries or injections, or both, are usually administered following transfer and for the following two weeks. If pregnancy does occur, you may be required to stay on these until you reach the twelve-week stage.

6. *Blastocyst transfer*

If you have had previous IVF failures, if your medical history indicates that there is a high chance of IVF failure this time, or if you have several good embryos on day 3, your doctor may recommend letting your embryos grow to blastocyst stage before transferring them. This usually occurs on day 5 after egg collection. Once an embryo reaches the blastocyst stage, it is ready for implantation. Transferring the embryo at this stage gives a greater chance of pregnancy. Not all Irish clinics offer a five-day transfer.

On day 4, the separate cells of the embryo start compressing together and become connected: this process is called compaction. When they are completely compacted, a tight ball is formed and no individual cells are evident. At this stage, the embryo is called a morula. On day 5, the morula pulls in fluid and begins to expand out like a bubble. Once a fluid-filled cavity is established, the embryo is called a blastocyst. It is now ready for implantation and should begin hatching out of its outer shell by the end of day 6.

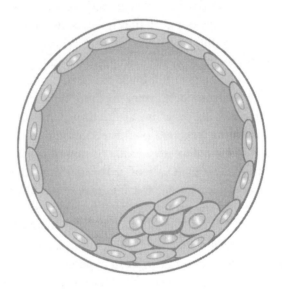

Fig. 7.2 Blastocyst

However, there is a risk associated with blastocyst culture: that is that the embryo will not make it to day 5. Only between 25 percent and 50 percent of embryos progress to the blastocyst stage after five days of culture. So you may end up with nothing to transfer; even if you do have something to transfer, you are likely to end up with fewer embryos, if any, to freeze.

7. *Frozen embryo transfer* (FET)

The term 'frozen embryos' refers to those embryos that were not transferred during an IVF cycle. The process of freezing embryos is known as embryo cryopreservation. These embryos can be thawed and then transferred into the uterus. Pregnancy rates are slightly lower for FETs than for fresh embryo transfers. The reason for this is that the highest-quality embryos are usually transferred immediately during the fresh cycle, and the ones that are frozen are usually of lesser quality. The success rate for FETs is about 15 to 20 percent, compared to 25 to 30 percent for fresh transfers.

There are three reasons why couples may undergo an FET:

    i.   There were embryos left over after a fresh transfer cycle.

    ii.   The fresh transfer was cancelled after the eggs were collected, and all resulting embryos were frozen. (This can be due to the risk of OHSS.)

    iii.   Donor embryos are being used.

Your body can be prepared for a FET in a number of ways. Your doctor may suggest going with your natural menstrual cycle, whereby your cycle will be monitored and the embryo transfer occurs a few days after ovulation. However, it is more common for ovulation to be shut down in a similar manner to preparation for a fresh cycle, and the uterine lining can then be prepared for the arrival of the embryos. Oestrogen supplements, in the form of tablets, patches, pessaries or injections, are administered in order to thicken the uterine lining.

Prior to transfer, your embryos will be thawed out. About 50 to 80 percent of embryos survive this thawing. The embryos can also be grown for a few days prior to transfer, if your doctor feels that you might benefit from having them grow to blastocyst stage.

The transfer itself is exactly like a fresh-embryo transfer. You will also probably be given progesterone supplementation afterwards.

8. *The two-week wait*

Apart from the medication protocol that your doctor has prescribed, there are a number of dos and don'ts for the 2ww. Each clinic may advise slightly differently; this is the advice I was given:

    i.   No intercourse

    ii.   Plenty of rest

    iii.   No heavy lifting or carrying

    iv.   No aerobic exercise

    v.   No hot baths, jacuzzis or saunas

Your clinic will give you an official test date, which is around fourteen days after transfer. They know that you will probably test sooner, but they will still want to know the result on your official test date.

Other tips, treatments and helpful advice

Apart from the medical steps involved, there are many alternative treatments that may help you get through the various steps of your cycle. I have also gathered a wealth of advice and information from couples who have already been through the process.

Before you start

You may be considering some alternative treatments to complement your IVF cycle. This can be for medical reasons or simply to help you relax. Acupuncture an hour or two before embryo transfer has been shown to improve pregnancy rates. It does this by using points that relax the uterus and improve the blood supply to it, thus promoting implantation. Acupuncture and reflexology can also be done throughout your IVF cycle (prior to egg collection) to aid relaxation: anything that helps you to relax during your cycle is helpful.

Nina Liu of Melt in Temple Bar suggests that clients do acupuncture for two to three months before they start IVF medication, in order to balance the body. She also highly recommends regular acupuncture around the time of egg collection and embryo transfer. She explains that this improves pregnancy rates because it builds your system and rebalances it after it has been disrupted by the IVF drugs. She says that you need to increase your kidney yang and rebalance your kidney yin; then when your body has been rebalanced, you have a much better chance of pregnancy.

Another consideration before you begin your cycle is whether or not to tell others your dates. While it can be of some comfort that those close to you know what you are going through, and when you are going through it, you may also feel some added pressure if others are constantly asking you about your cycle, especially towards the end of the 2ww. Some people suggest telling others that your test date is a week or two after the official one: that way, you have time to come to terms with a bad result before having to talk about it with others.

1. *Downregulation*

You need to start taking regular medication at this stage. A good way to make sure you don't forget is to set an alarm on your phone at appropriate intervals.

Take it easy at this stage: it can be a fairly relaxing time, as you are on your way, yet there is not much to do. I found it a bit of a relief to be off the TTC treadmill for a while. There is little chance of conceiving while you are shutting down your ovaries, so there is nothing to obsess about on a day-to-day basis!

2. *Ovarian stimulation*

Again, set alarms on your phone to remind you to take your medication.

Drink plenty of water to prevent OHSS and constipation. Your clinic will probably advise you to drink at least one and a half litres of water per day from the start of stimulation. If you are not used to drinking water, this can be a full-time job, with toilet trips every quarter of an hour until your body gets used to the volume of liquid! You may find it easier to start a week or two beforehand and build up to one and a half litres a day. After about a week, your body will be more used to the volume of water, and the frequency of toilet trips will subside.

Many people advise eating plenty of protein, to aid the growth of cells in your eggs. It certainly won't do any harm. This recipe is healthy, yummy and full of protein:

IVF protein smoothie
  Quinoa or rice milk
  1 serving spirulina
  2 tablespoons ground mixed seed
      (pumpkin, sunflower, hemp, linseed)
  1 teaspoon calcium/magnesium/zinc powder
  1 tablespoon hemp-seed oil
  Fruit or veg as desired
      (I used frozen summer berries, available from supermarkets)

Take one smoothie a day from the start of stims, to aid egg production. A word of warning: you need to drink more water to compensate for the seeds, as they will add bulk to your large intestine and can cause you to become constipated.

Ask your doctor what vitamins and supplements may be suitable for you. Many women take Vitamin C and B12 for general well-being. Folic acid is essential at this stage to prevent neural-tube defects in your baby; it should be started three months before conception.

Avoid overheating during stimulation. Your doctor will probably advise against aerobic exercise: don't forget that this can include hoovering! Men: this is where you finally get to play a part in things!

3. *Egg collection*

You will definitely need someone to come with you, or at least to drop you off and pick you up, as you will feel very sleepy afterwards. You will probably be advised not to drive for twenty-four hours.

When you get home, continue to drink plenty of water, as OHSS is still a risk at this stage, even if you haven't shown signs of it before.

Nina from Melt advises that it is very important to watch what you eat around egg collection and embryo transfer. She says that you should try to take in more warm food and less cold food, in order to increase your kidney yang. She suggests foods such as lamb stew, sweet potatoes and sweetcorn.

4. *Fertilisation*

For many, the wait for the fertilisation report is the most stressful time of the whole cycle. Try to ensure that whichever of you is due to get the call is not alone that day, as staring at a phone for eight hours can test the best of us. Plan lots of nice things for both of you to do during the two to five days between egg collection and embryo transfer, to try and take your minds off things. At this stage, your work is done and you have to put your trust in the embryologist.

5. *Embryo transfer*

Research shows that acupuncture an hour or two before embryo transfer can improve pregnancy rates. Some suggest that another treatment an hour or two afterwards helps further. Because you may not know the exact time and date of your transfer until a day or two beforehand, make sure that your acupuncturist is flexible enough to fit you in when you need it. If you think there may be a problem, try someone else who can guarantee your treatment. You will have enough to worry about without fretting that you won't be able to get your acupuncture at the right time.

Do not fill your bladder too much before you get to the clinic: it is easy to drink a little more when you get there, but much harder to pee a little out. I drank the full one and a half litres as recommended before I left the house and was in agony at the clinic for about half an hour before a nurse advised me to go and pee a little out. Many people recommend not drinking any water before you get to the clinic, as it takes only around twenty minutes for your bladder to fill up.

Don't forget to ask your doctor or nurse if they saw the flash. You may even get a picture of it.

6. *Blastocyst transfer*

This is the most stressful procedure of all, as there is always a chance that no embryos will make it to this stage. All I can advise is to keep yourselves busy at this time and check in regularly with your clinic for updates.

7. *Frozen-embryo transfer*

As the transfer itself is the same as a fresh transfer, the same advice applies here.

8. *The 2ww*

Many people suggest eating fresh pineapple from the time of embryo transfer to promote implantation. TCM advises keeping your feet warm to aid implantation.

As for dealing with the emotional side of the 2ww, I wish I knew how to do it! It has helped me to talk to others online who are going through the same thing at the same time as me. However, you take the chance that you might be the one left behind at the end of it. When it comes to testing, I have always been one to test early and often. It breaks me in gently, gives me something to do, and prevents the short, sharp shock of a definitive 'no' at the end of the cycle. However, this does not work for everyone, and many prefer to put off testing for as long as possible. If you have come this far, you probably already know what works best for you. Good luck!

What are the risks involved?

The main risk involved with IVF is the risk that it will not work. For many, IVF is considered their last chance of having a baby – the treatment they would always have to fall back on if all else failed. It may not work the first time – or the second or third time. Your age and infertility diagnosis will give you a better idea of your odds, but even women in their twenties with no fertility issues have failed IVF cycles. Unfortunately, there is no stock advice I can give you at this point. A failed IVF cycle (or one that is cancelled or results in miscarriage) is a devastating experience for anyone and is impossible to prepare for adequately. Different couples have different ways of facing the possibility of failure. I dealt with it by ensuring that, as much as was possible, I had the details of my next cycle lined up in advance. Others try not to think about failure, relying on hope to get them through the cycle. Obviously we all have hope that we will get pregnant, otherwise we wouldn't be doing IVF in the first place, but how you deal with the balance of hope and disappointment is a personal decision.

The main physical risk of IVF is that the ovaries may become over-stimulated, resulting in OHSS (see page 135). Your doctor will advise you on your personal risk given your age and medical history, and will also advise you on the steps you need to take to reduce this risk. You need to be vigilant for any possible symptoms of OHSS and you should also drink plenty of water: at least one and a half litres a day from the start of stimulation is advisable, and up to three litres if you can manage it.

On the other side of the coin, there is the risk that your ovaries will not respond adequately (and sometimes not at all) to stimulation, and that you will not produce enough follicles to go ahead with egg collection. The number of follicles that is considered adequate depends on your clinic and your own infertility circumstances. Usually, egg collection is not considered worthwhile unless there are at least three or four follicles, but pregnancies have been achieved with only one follicle. (I achieved a pregnancy with three mature follicles, which produced two eggs.) If it is your first cycle, your doctor may advise you to try again with a different protocol, thus saving you the expense and physical hardship of a cycle that has a slim chance of success. However, if you have responded poorly to stimulation in the past, if you have had several previous failed cycles, or if you are over forty, another cycle may not produce any better results, and you may be advised to go ahead with egg collection.

There is also the risk of multiples. While it is most infertiles' dream to get 'two for the price of one', you should be aware of the risks associated with twin and triplet pregnancies. The chance of miscarriage is higher than with a singleton pregnancy, as is the risk of preterm delivery. The mother also has a greater risk of high blood pressure, pre-eclampsia, gestational diabetes, anaemia and caesarean section.

What are the success rates?

Success rates for IVF depend largely on the age of the woman and the cause of infertility. For the under-thirty-fives, pregnancy rates can be as high as 40 percent. This decreases steadily after the age of thirty-five, with less than 10 percent of cycles resulting in pregnancy by the age of forty-three. Overall, success rates are between 25 and 30 percent; this falls to 15 to 20 percent for FETs. However, success rates for those using donor eggs are around 65 percent across all ages. This is because the chances of success depend on the age of the donor, not the recipient.

Louise from Dublin

In May 2004, after trying to conceive for nearly two years, we finally found out what was wrong: Robert's sperm count was extremely low. It wasn't a huge surprise, as he had had undescended testes as a child. Once we knew this and had got our referral to the Rotunda HARI unit, things started to move quite quickly for us. Male-factor seemed to be easier to treat than female- or unknown-factor infertility, and the HARI unit were optimistic about our chances, seeing as I was under thirty.

Unfortunately, there were initial hold-ups before we could start IVF: very frustratingly, my smear test came back with abnormal cells, which needed to be burnt off. This set us back about six months. It was the most maddening thing for me: I just wanted to go ahead and was sick of being in limbo. Funnily enough, I didn't care at all about the abnormal cells, just that it was delaying our chance of having a baby!

I found the cycle of IVF fine. People at work were very good about giving me time off, and I was so delighted to be able to have the IVF and to be doing something positive towards having a baby that I went in to all the appointments smiling and came out of egg collection laughing.

The dreaded two-week wait turned out to be only a dreaded one-week wait. A few days after embryo transfer, I began to feel very

---

bloated: none of my jeans would fit me. At one stage, in work, I remember going into the kitchen and lying down on the floor – which was the only relief I could find from the pressure. Eventually, I went into HARI and they admitted me straight away, with OHSS. I remember the doctor storming into the ward and snapping at one of the nurses: 'Why hasn't a test been done. You don't get this without pregnancy.' But I didn't dare hope. The nurse drew my blood, all the time reminding me that it was very early, and I could get a false negative. My husband arrived in. Two other ladies who were in the ward recovering from hysterectomies very kindly left the room so we could have some privacy. The nurse came back in. I couldn't read her face, then she broke into a big smile and said: 'It's positive.' It turned out to be twins!

Susan from Limerick

I was one of the naive ones who never in a million years thought I'd need IVF. Our daughter was conceived the old-fashioned way, but when we started trying again, we were faced with lots of heartache and problems before I was finally referred for treatment. Secondary infertility is kind of a weird place where you don't really belong anywhere. You should be thankful for what you have, and yet . . . .

For those of you on the assisted-conception journey: be prepared for the waiting. Depending on the clinic you go to, you might have to wait quite some time to start, and us 'elder lemons' (in fertility terms) really need to get cracking quickly to increase our chances of success! Delays are not good, and clinics vary in how they approach starting treatment.

Be prepared to be cancelled at your first scan, no matter how healthy or otherwise glib you might feel about your prospects. Have your partner with you just in case. I didn't, and was devastated all by myself in the car park of the Rotunda. Not good.

Be prepared to move clinics if you are needlessly delayed. Nice and empathetic as the clinic staff can be, sometimes a different approach is needed. Do your homework, and be decisive.

Be prepared for a big shock when you see the size of the pack of medication, never mind the array of syringes and needles. Even though I knew the pack would be hefty, it was a shock when I got home and opened up all the packets and found my bed festooned with a scary range of paraphernalia. The horror of it all – realising that I would have to shove all these drugs into me over a few weeks, with no guarantees – took a while for me to get my head around.

Initially, I was very open with family and close friends, and asked for their prayers and good wishes. However, while my mum and sister in particular were incredibly supportive and wanted to know all the details (which I shared during my first cycle), I did find it very draining having to constantly explain all the nitty-gritty, as they just didn't understand what I was going through. Eventually, I was quite vague, as I found it quite pressurising to have my fertility – or lack of it – be the focus of everyone's attention. On my final cycle, I told absolutely no one, and it was incredibly liberating.

That Christmas Eve, we were able to tell our daughter that she would be a big sister after waiting seven long years, and the next summer, the waiting and constant worry finally ended when I heard my little boy cry. Words simply cannot describe the profound joy of that sound.

He is a miracle boy, and the product of much sadness, determination and optimism, tempered with realism, drugs and pain – but mostly hope.

IVF with ICSI (Intracytoplasmic Sperm Injection)

ICSI involves the injection of a single sperm into the egg. It is a very effective method of fertilisation, with about a fertilisation rate of 70 to 85 percent, compared to about 66 percent without ICSI.

Who might benefit?

Couples with severe male-factor infertility (i.e. those with very low sperm counts, motility or morphology) are usually advised to try ICSI when the sperm is not considered to be of a high enough quality or quantity to achieve normal fertilisation rates on its own. Couples who have had no, or low, fertilisation rates on previous IVF cycles may benefit from ICSI. Also, couples with a low yield of eggs at egg collection may benefit from ICSI, as it has a slightly higher fertilisation rate than IVF on its own.

What is the cost?

As ICSI is part of the IVF process, all the associated costs of IVF apply. ICSI costs approximately €1,000 on top of the costs of IVF; again, this is not covered by any Irish health insurers.

What does it involve?

In order to inject the sperm into the egg, the egg is held with a special pipette. A very delicate, sharp, hollow needle is used to immobilise and pick up a single sperm. The needle is then carefully inserted through the hard shell of the egg and into the cytoplasm. The sperm is injected into the cytoplasm, and the needle is removed. The sperm is then left to fertilise the egg.

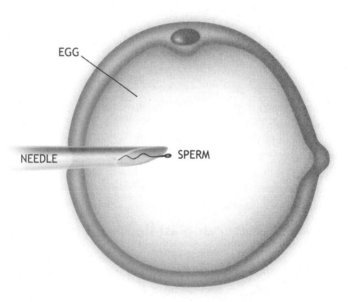

Fig. 7.3 ICSI (Intracytoplasmic Sperm Injection)

What are the success rates?

Fertilisation rates are usually 70 to 85 percent. Some studies have found that pregnancy rates are slightly higher in IVF with ICSI than without it. However, this may be because, in many cases of male-factor infertility, the woman does not have any fertility problems; as a result, once viable embryos are transferred, pregnancy is more likely.

Preimplantation Genetic Diagnosis – PGD

PGD is a technique that was developed in the 1980s as a means of testing embryos for genetic disorders before transferring the embryos to the woman's uterus. It involves removing a cell from an embryo at the eight-cell stage (usually on day 3) and testing it for specific genetic information. At this stage of development, all of the embryo cells are identical and have yet to develop their own specialist functions. Because of this, the removal of one cell does not damage the embryo's ability to continue developing normally.

PGD is not currently permitted in Ireland and many couples travel abroad to avail of it. However, the Commission on Assisted Human Reproduction (CAHR) report of 2005 has recommended that PGD should be allowed in Ireland, under regulation, in order to reduce the risk of serious genetic disorders. In the UK, the use of PGD is allowed to check embryos for certain conditions such as cystic fibrosis and Huntington's disease, and also for genes that significantly increase the risk of certain cancers. The UK also allows embryos to be selected on the basis that they are a tissue match for a sick sibling.

The use of PGD is controversial, not least because some countries allow its use for gender selection. The 2005 CAHR report recommends that sex selection should be permitted in Ireland but only for the reliable prevention of serious sex-linked genetic disorders and not for social reasons.

Donor sperm and eggs

Donor sperm has been used in fertility treatment in the USA since the 1920s and in the UK for the last forty years. It was introduced in Ireland in 1980. As yet, there are no laws governing the provision of ART services (including those using donor gametes) in Ireland, but there are guidelines for doctors issued by the Irish Medical Council. There are approximately 250 babies conceived by donor sperm born each year in Ireland, and six clinics offer IUI and IVF with donor sperm:

Sims Clinic, Dublin – *www.simsclinic.ie*

Clane Hospital, County Kildare – *www.clanehospital.ie*

Kilkenny – *www.thekilkennyclinic.com*

Cork Fertility Centre – (021) 486 5764

Galway – (091) 544 223

Morehampton Clinic (IUI only) – *www.infertility.ie*

Alison from Dublin

The decision to use donor sperm was very difficult for us in the beginning. We just weren't sure if we were doing the right thing. In the end, we both just wanted a baby, and I knew my husband would make a wonderful father. We had all the right ingredients to make a baby; all we were missing was good sperm. The donor process gave us the gift of being able to experience conception and pregnancy, which we both decided was very important to us.

After a long struggle with IUI and then with IVF, we made our baby together. My husband gave me the injections and was there with me every step of the way. We are watching my belly grow together and are as excited as we could possibly be at the prospect of meeting our son. Using a donor is not for everyone, but it was definitely the right decision for us.

The Sims Clinic in Dublin was the first Irish clinic to offer IVF with donor eggs. There is more information on the programme they offer at *www.eggdonation.ie*. The Cork Fertility Centre also offers a donor-egg service, but this is usually with a donor who is known to the couple receiving treatment. The Kilkenny Clinic, Clane Hospital and the Galway Fertility Unit do an initial consultation for egg donation and then refer patients to clinics abroad. They will also do any monitoring that needs to be done while patients are in Ireland.

Only one Irish clinic, the Morehampton Clinic in Dublin, currently offers ART treatments to single women and lesbian couples, as previous Irish Medical Council guidelines advised against this. However, the Commission on Assisted Human Reproduction (CAHR) report of 2005 recommends that ART services should be available without discrimination on the grounds of gender, marital status or sexual orientation, so this situation may change in the future.

At present, sperm or egg donors have the right to anonymity in Ireland, should they so wish. It is up to you to decide whether you would prefer to use a known or an anonymous donor. There is a much wider availability of gametes from anonymous donors. However, the right to anonymity by a donor was removed in the UK in 2005, and the CAHR report of 2005 recommended that any child born through the use of donated gametes or embryos should, on maturity, be allowed to identify the donor (or donors) involved in his or her conception. While this may be the ideal situation for some, there is a risk that the availability of donor gametes could be seriously reduced should this become law.

The decision whether or not, and when, to tell your child about the manner of his or her conception requires very careful consideration and should be discussed at length with a counsellor before any decisions are made. You may also wish to talk to other couples about their experiences. The UK-based Donor Conception Network can provide support and information on this topic:

www.donor-conception-network.org
PO Box 7471, Nottingham NG3 6ZR
+44 208 245 4369

Egg freezing

Egg freezing, or oocyte cryopreservation, is a relatively new and developing technology. It is currently only available in Ireland to cancer patients who may be left infertile by their treatment. To date, a slow-freezing method has been used, and this has a relatively low success rate: only 50 to 60 percent of eggs survive the thaw. A new rapid-freeze process, known as vitrification, claims to give eggs a 90 to 95 percent chance of survival. The Sims Clinic in Dublin is considering introducing this service, and several UK clinics already offer it.

A legal perspective on fertility treatment in Ireland

ART services in Ireland are not currently subject to any statutory control. There is no law preventing IVF, but there is no legal framework regulating it either. However, there are ethical guidelines issued by the Irish Medical Council (see *www.medicalcouncil.ie*).

A Commission on Assisted Human Reproduction was established by the government in 2000 to prepare a report to recommend a legal framework for assisted reproduction. The report was completed in April 2005 and is available from the Department of Health and Children (*www.dohc.ie*). There have, as yet, been no policy decisions made as a result of this report.

ART services are not available on the public-health service in Ireland, and no health insurers cover IUI or IVF costs. You can, however, claim tax relief on all expenses using the MED1 form, which is available from *www.revenue.ie*. The HARI Clinic at the Rotunda does fund a few places for public patients, but the waiting list is very long. The Merrion Fertility Clinic at Holles Street and the Galway Fertility Clinic at the University Hospital take medical-card patients at a discounted rate.

All medication for ART is covered under the Drugs Payment Scheme, which ensures that no individual or family in Ireland has to pay more than €90 per month in prescription charges. There is more information on this scheme at *www.citizensinformation.ie*.

8

Surviving infertility

Introduction

One in six Irish couples trying to conceive will not do so on their own. Infertility is the label given to those couples who have not managed to conceive after twelve months of well-timed intercourse, or after six months if the woman is over thirty-five. It is also sometimes applied to couples who have not been able to carry a baby to term. It is a label that is very hard for some couples to accept, even if they are willing to concede that they may need help. If you don't want to call yourselves infertile, then don't: you can say that you are having problems conceiving, or that you need a bit of medical intervention to have a baby. Surviving this difficult time is all about doing what is best for you, and identifying the ways in which the emotional baggage can be minimised. Different approaches work for different people, and in the end it is up to you to decide what you can cope with, and what will help make your lives more bearable.

Nobody starts out on their TTC journey expecting to get to this stage. Most couples who decide to have a baby together have been used to taking steps to prevent pregnancy, and assume that, once they have stopped using contraception, pregnancy will soon follow. Six to twelve months is a very long time to spend getting your hopes up and having them knocked down on a regular basis. If you have not already done so, it is time to seek help. Chapter 5 can point you in the direction of medical treatment to overcome your physical problems, but what about the emotional turmoil that infertility brings?

There is no easy answer. It is extremely difficult not to compare yourselves to other couples and agonise over why this is happening to you. Sadly though, it *is* happening, and you need to find ways of coping, because the one sure-fire way of not getting pregnant is to give up and stop getting up in the mornings! This chapter will bring you through the small steps of dealing with a failed cycle, to the larger steps of sharing the burden with others and helping them to help you.

Dealing with a failed cycle

This section is for those with fairly regular, ovulatory cycles. For those with very irregular or lengthy cycles, there is more information in Chapters 2, 3, 5 and 6.

A cycle fails in different ways for different people. Some people hold out on testing and wait for their period to arrive. Even if the tell-tale signs have been there, the onset of a period can be a big shock, as there is almost no hope of pregnancy once any sort of bleeding begins. Other people will test at 12, 13 or 14 DPO (days past ovulation); while a negative test at this stage is not a definitive indication that this cycle has failed to result in a pregnancy, it is unlikely that the outcome will be positive, and again this can feel like a kick in the guts. If you are charting your temperature (see Chapter 3), you may prefer to hold off testing and wait for a temperature drop. This doesn't necessarily mean that you are out of the running, but it is a very good indicator that your period is on the way. Again, this is an instant disappointment.

I take the unenviable approach of starting testing as soon as it is physically possible to have seen a rise in HCG levels (the level of pregnancy hormone in your body – see Chapter 2). In fact, I am going to own up and admit to testing even earlier than that at times.

As implantation takes place from about 7 DPO (see Chapter 2), the very earliest you can expect to see any sort of a test line on a home-pregnancy test is 8 DPO – and that is if you are testing with the most sensitive tests on the market (see Chapter 2). I have to say that I do not recommend testing this early, and if you can possibly hold out until 10 DPO, then please do. Testing early and seeing a negative result only increases the period of 'mourning' for a failed cycle by an extra few days. However, the one benefit of this approach is that it eases you into disappointment rather than leaving you with one big shock at the end of the cycle. A negative test at 8 DPO can be shrugged off with the confidence that it is probably too early; the same at 9 DPO. By 10 DPO, you can start to prepare yourself for another cycle, and by 12 DPO you will probably have got your head around the idea. Therefore, there is no one day of breakdown – but unfortunately several days of disappointment.

It is really up to you to decide which approach is less painful for you. You might feel that the short, sharp shock at the end of a cycle is preferable to the long, drawn-out rigmarole of daily testing. My decision is driven by my desire to know about a pregnancy as soon as possible; I have tried alternative approaches, but they just didn't work for me. The fact of the matter is that none of us likes to think that a cycle is definitely going to fail, no matter how difficult the circumstances. In the end, we always hope for a miracle, otherwise why would we bother? However, given that optimism precedes any given cycle, we must prepare ourselves to deal with the outcome in a way that limits the inevitable pain of failure.

So whether your worst day is day 1 of your cycle, or your first realistic negative test, there are four steps you can take to avoid meltdown:

1. Allow yourself one day of mourning

Firstly, cry. And cry and cry and cry and cry. Cry as much or as little as you need to. Don't feel like you are the only person in the world to wail uncontrollably at the end of the cycle; there are women (and sometimes men) doing the same thing at the same time as you, all over the country. Cry for the baby you won't get to hold in eight months' time, the sister who is heavily pregnant, the insensitive comments your best friend made, and just how bloody unfair it all is.

A good friend recommends one day of very bad behaviour (crying, screaming, drinking, wallowing in self-pity), and then that's it – one day is all that is allowed. This is very good advice, and everyone should give it a go if at all possible. Write it on a piece of paper and stick it on your fridge so you won't forget. You can allow yourself a few more days if you have had a failed treatment cycle.

2. This too shall pass

No matter how bad you feel, and no matter how hard you cry, you must call to mind the most important rule of surviving failed cycles: never forget that *this too shall pass*. Whether you count yourself out at 12 DPO or day 1 of your cycle, remember that this is the hardest day. You will not feel like this in a few days' time, and you will be ready to try again before long. My cycles tend to go like this:

CD (cycle day)1 to 2: Depression

CD 3 to 8: Start looking forward, thinking about ovulation

CD 9 to 15: Go, go, go catch that egg!

CD 15 to 18: Chart temp rise, pat myself on the back when I achieve coverline (see Chapter 3 on charting temperatures)

CD 19 to 22: Excitedly plan future with new baby

CD 23 to 25: Testing phase

I have been known to be as happy and carefree as a normal person from days nine to twenty-two; in fact, I can be positively radiant with expectation. While there is little consolation available at the start or the end of a cycle, you can aim to be at your best mid-cycle. Learn to recognise the emotional life cycle of your period so that you can plan social and family events for your good times – or even so that you can simply remember that there *are* good times.

3. Activate your back-up plan

It is very important to have a back-up plan. Although you may not want to contemplate the failure of a cycle while there is still hope, it is very advisable to have a Plan B to fall back on, just in case. Putting this structure in place before a cycle fails gives you something to concentrate on as soon as you realise that it has not been your month.

This back-up plan can be a medical one: if this cycle fails, then we will go to our GP, move on to a stronger dose of Clomid, investigate IVF, or whatever the next step might be. This puts the disappointment of a failed cycle in the context of a greater plan and can help you to keep looking forward.

Your back-up plan can also be a personal plan: a weekend away, say, or a course you've always wanted to do. I have infertility to thank for helping me learn Spanish – something I finally got around to organising in a bid to stop me wasting time I no longer spent socialising.

Breaking your TTC journey down into manageable steps also means that you can take one step at a time and concentrate on doing the best you can at that stage with the knowledge that is available to you. If investigations at any stage show that you need to move on to further stage, then you will arrive there fully prepared.

As long as you have something in the pipeline, something to look forward to, there is a reason to go on – with TTC and with life. And we can't forget about life in this great journey!

4. Buy yourself something you can't afford

Finally, treat yourself. Go on, buy yourself something you can't afford. You deserve it. A new pair of boots – why not? I always go for the boots! Obviously not every month – sometimes it's just a simple item of make-up or a nice bottle of wine. Or even something nice for my lunch. This month I treated myself to pancakes and maple syrup for breakfast and I savoured every mouthful of it. Next month, more boots!

Putting yourself first

Infertility is a tough battle. You have to grin and bear the consequences of each failed cycle, every pregnancy announcement, every cute and funny anecdote about your colleague's baby. So give yourselves a break and limit the damage. Just say no! Forget about your cousin's daughter's christening, don't feel obliged to attend the friend's dinner party that coincides with the arrival of your period. They don't need you to be there: they might like you to be, but the show will still go on without you. A basic rule of thumb is that if you think you will spend more time worrying about the function than you will enjoying it, then it is best to send your regrets early on. If you feel up to it, let your friend or cousin know why it will be too hard for you to attend. If not, don't worry about it: people turn down invitations all the time. Most importantly, don't beat yourself up about doing the 'right' thing. The right thing is for you to look after yourself, and to do what makes you happy. Or at least what makes you least miserable.

Coping with important dates

There are always dates that we deem significant – six months trying, a year trying, a miscarried baby's due date or anniversary. How many times have you prayed to be pregnant by Christmas, new year, or your birthday? If a date is important to you, then mark it in whatever way you want. If you want to take the day off and spend it with your partner, then don't feel bad pulling a sickie or using a holiday. If you want to spend the day under your duvet, well go ahead, we've all been there. (But remember, one day of mourning!) However, try to keep looking forward and focusing on your next step: an upcoming doctor's appointment or treatment cycle. That way, the significant date does not have to be the end of a chapter, just another part of the story.

Coping with festive occasions

Festive occasions can be the most difficult times of the year. Christmas, your birthday, Mother's Day, Father's Day – they all serve to remind you of what you don't have, and what you have lost during the year. There is no easy way to get through these times, and you certainly can't make your infertility disappear for the day, but if you are prepared, then you can minimise the stress, and maybe even enjoy yourselves a little.

Accepting that Christmas, birthdays and other festive occasions will not be easy, and taking steps to prepare for this, is half the battle. Burying your head in the sand and refusing to acknowledge that Christmas is coming will not make it go away. If you can plan events that you can do together, avoiding functions that may upset you, then you will have a reason to get excited about the festive period. Organise a trip to the theatre, a special meal just for the two of you, a weekend away – whatever you both like to do the most. Just make sure that you have something to look forward to.

However you choose to mark your birthday, Christmas Day or even Mother's Day, remember that it is only one day. After twenty-four hours, it will be over, and life will return to 'normal'. And hopefully the next festive occasion will be very different.

Getting help

Whether or not you have the support of friends and family, it can be very liberating to discuss your feelings about infertility with people who are going through the same process, or with a counsellor who is trained in helping couples deal with the emotional effects of infertility.

Online support groups

The first port of call for many is the Internet. For those with a computer and Internet access, it is the easiest way of finding out how others cope with infertility. Chapter 4 takes you through the basics of getting online, finding others in the same boat, and learning the lingo of TTC. It also lists useful TTC websites, message boards and blogs, both in Ireland and abroad. You can visit those sites or find your own, browse a little, lurk a little, or post a few messages to find the site that suits you best. You may wish to join a local online message board in the hope of finding people you can meet and chat to in real life, or you may prefer to preserve your anonymity and join an American site, for example, for online support only.

Internet message boards can foster a real sense of community, and can be a life-saver for those who have little real-life support. They can also be a great source of information, and you can be sure to pick up all the info on the latest TTC trends. How else would I have found out that taking cough medicine increases cervical mucus? Or that an increase in cervical mucus is to be desired?

When you join a message board, it is likely that most people are at the same stage of TTC. If you join a group for people who have been trying for over a year, then most people will probably be at the one- to two-year stage. Some, maybe most, of those people will go on to become pregnant; hopefully you will be one of them. But what if you are not? What if you have to face one pregnancy announcement after another, until your brave face becomes too hard to wear?

I would not have got to where I am now without the support I have found on the Internet. I have made friendships with women from all over the world, and have become good friends with a few locally too. I have kept myself informed and updated constantly, and regularly seek support and solace at my computer. However, the ease with which we can access information and support online does not come without a price. Online chat rooms and message boards can become addictive, and can eat into time that might be better spent with family and friends. Does my online support help me get through the day? Yes. Does it distract me from other things that might help me get through the day? Yes. In the end, it is about recognising that life outside of infertility goes on, whether you like it or not, and that, if you're not careful, it might just pass you by.

Local support groups

If you would prefer to meet up with other infertile women or couples without meeting them online first, then the National Infertility Support and Information Group (NISIG) can put you in touch with your local group. As well as infertility support groups, NISIG has groups that discuss donor conception and living life without children. You can reach them online at *www.infertilityireland.ie* or you can call them on 1890 647 444. NISIG produces a regular newsletter for members; this contains information about local meetings and articles, and news about infertility. These newsletters are also available from your fertility clinic.

Counselling services

Many people find it helpful to be able to talk about their problems in an environment where they can let all their emotions out, and where they will be listened to without judgement. If you would like to talk to someone in confidence, your fertility clinic can put you in touch with someone who is trained in dealing with infertility issues. If you have not yet got to the fertility-clinic stage, you can contact NISIG (contact details above). You may also ask your GP, although you should check to make sure that your GP's recommended counsellor has experience of dealing with infertility. Sometimes a counsellor who does not know the right things to say can be worse than no counsellor at all. If you are not happy with your counsellor – because they have no experience of dealing with infertility, or for any other reason – don't feel obliged to see them again. It is of the utmost importance that you are comfortable with your counsellor and confident about speaking to him or her. If you are not able to build up a relationship of trust, then you are better off seeking help elsewhere, either with an alternative counsellor or via one of the other channels discussed here.

Men and infertility

Infertility is too often seen as a 'woman's issue', both from a physical and an emotional point of view. It is seen as the woman's task to monitor her fertility, watch out for ovulation and deal with a failed cycle. Even if a couple suffers from male-factor infertility, most of the treatment, literature and support is directed towards the female partner. This can distance men from the day-to-day reality of infertility, and they may feel that their only role is to comfort their partner in times of need.

Our society views women first and foremost as mothers; it does not hold fatherhood in the same regard. Despite the fact that you and your partner may want exactly the same things for your family, it may be difficult for you to understand the drive and depth of feeling she has towards having a baby. You may feel pushed aside at times, while her grief seems to take priority over your own.

It is normal not to feel as devastated as your partner at the end of each cycle. Don't feel inadequate because your tears are no match for hers. Don't forget that, apart from the disappointment and pain of not being pregnant yet again, she has probably worked herself up into a frenzy, monitoring every ache and twinge for signs of pregnancy: the stress of that alone can cause some hangover at the start of a new cycle. Regardless of the medical problem that is preventing you from conceiving, it is your partner who will have to undergo endless procedures and treatments. As she is constantly talking to her doctors and her support network, she will be very well informed about the investigations and treatments she is having, and the drugs she is taking. As none of this is happening to you, it is understandable that your eyes may glaze over at the mention of another supplement or procedure. Even if the subject bores you to tears, try to feign interest: your partner will appreciate it, even though she will probably see right through your feeble attempts to appear fascinated by what she is saying!

You may feel anger and frustration at the way in which your lives have changed. You might look at your partner and be sad to have lost the woman you fell for – and wish that you could do anything to get her back. You will most likely blame infertility for doing this to you, and it is very easy to lose sight of the reason you embarked on this journey in the first place. If you feel this happening, it is time for a break. Treat your partner to a night out or a weekend away – on the condition that you keep the amount of time you spend talking about infertility to a minimum. It will do you the world of good to remember why you are on this journey, and why you fell in love in the first place.

It is rare to find men posting on the parenting websites that are listed in Chapter 4, but it does happen occasionally, and the women there tend to be very impressed – and more than happy to help out. There is also a small, but growing, community of male infertility bloggers that you might be interested in checking out:

www.offsprung.blogspot.com
www.smarshyboy.blogspot.com
www.malefactorinfertility.blogspot.com
www.dadsomeday.blogspot.com

Talking to family and friends

Many people prefer to keep their infertility to themselves, finding it easier to get on with life without those around them knowing what they are going through. Others choose to have their problems out in the open – at least to some extent – as it can be very difficult to put a brave face on all the time. Only you can decide how you want to deal with the situation. While it can help to have family and friends around at the most difficult times, the compromise is that your trials and treatments will spill over into other areas of your life, and sometimes it can feel like there is little more to you than infertility.

I have chosen to be out of the closet pretty much from the start of our TTC journey. It began when we married, so we knew that there would be plenty of pairs of eyes looking in our direction. I also made no secret of my desire to have several more children, and having conceived our son without any problems, I saw no problems in declaring that there would be another one on the way before long.

My struggle for another child has become my life. I still work, I still socialise, but I am very aware that people either make a concerted effort to ask me how I am (i.e. are you pregnant yet?) or completely avoid the issue. This is something that I can bear, as I would have found it impossible to carry on with life without being able to explain what is going on in my head and why I may not be acting quite like myself some of the time. It also allows me to turn down invitations to potentially difficult social events with the simple reply: 'Sorry, but that would be too hard for me right now.'

Whether you have been open from the start, or have come to a point in your journey where you feel it would be helpful to share your experiences with a loved one, there are some issues you might need to consider.

Taking the first steps

Talking to family and friends about your infertility can be a challenging and frustrating experience. Unless your friend or family member has experience of infertility, either first hand or through someone close to them, it is unlikely that they will have any idea of how much you are hurting.

It is impossible for others to put themselves in your shoes. They may have children already, or they may want them at some stage in the future, or maybe they have no plans to have children. Whatever their situation, it is difficult for them to understand how painful it can be to tell people that you are infertile.

I always wanted children – lots of them. Although infertility was one of my greatest fears, it was not something that bore heavily on me – at least only to the extent that I didn't want to put off having children for too long, just in case. I didn't know anyone who was infertile, so I could only guess at how hard it might be.

I didn't have a clue. My guess only extended to the long-term pain a couple might feel about not having a child in their lives. Many people, fuelled by inaccuracies contained in TV dramas, assume that there is a once-off diagnosis that a couple has to deal with, and that they are then free to return to their lives and reshape their future without their much-wanted child. If only it was that easy.

It is very difficult to explain the cumulative effect of month after month, and year after year, of disappointment, without making it look as though you are just not coping very well with TTC – something most people breeze through. Now matter how much that person cares about you, this is probably new territory for them, and it is useful to have some answers prepared for the questions they are likely to ask. Only you can decide how much detail you want to share, how much intrusion you can deal with, and how much this person is likely to help ease your burden.

1. Decide how much information you wish to share

This is something you need to discuss with each other before sharing information with family and friends. It is often the case that the woman has become so accustomed to talking to doctors and her support network about the workings of her reproductive system that she will share this information with family and friends without a second thought. On the other hand, her partner may not be so eager to tell all about his low sperm count or the fact that he had to have a 'quick one' in a doctor's office.

Even if you are happy to talk about the procedures and treatments you have been through, you may choose to keep the results to yourself. However, most people seem to assume that the 'fault' lies with the woman, and may offer advice, such as to take certain supplements, eat fish or do yoga. As 35 percent of couples with problems suffer exclusively from male-factor infertility (35 percent is female-factor, 20 percent a combination, and 10 percent unexplained), this sort of unsolicited advice can be highly irritating. It is up to you how much you can take!

2. Plan what you're going to say

As your loved one is unlikely to have any idea what you have been going through, it is very important to choose your words carefully. Unless this person is highly skilled in dealing with sensitive emotional issues, it is likely that either they won't know what to say, or they will say the wrong thing. Even the most caring friend may offer a suggestion that sounds wildly insensitive to you. You need to do your best to anticipate their responses and prepare carefully worded answers to their likely questions.

Many people feel as though they have to say something when bad or sad news is shared with them. They might feel that some words of consolation are better than none. They may also mistakenly assume that you are looking for advice rather than comfort and support.

As I am very open about our own situation, I constantly find myself dealing with platitudes and unsolicited advice. Before I had a list of witty and informative repartees up my sleeve, I often found myself getting upset and frustrated trying to explain to people why just relaxing or taking a holiday wasn't going to help us – which only served to fuel their belief that I really did need to relax or go on holiday. It is not enough to tell people that relaxing does not help infertile couples, as it is an untruth universally accepted that this is indeed the case.

If your loved one advises you to relax, eat more fish or go on a cruise, you need to explain calmly, and with as much medical evidence as you can find in advance, why this will not work for you. Stanton's 2002 article[1] explains that researchers have confirmed that biomedical causes account for most fertility problems. Anderheim's 2005 study[2] shows that the stress levels of IVF patients had no effect on pregnancy rates, while the 2000 study by Baik Seok Kee et al[3] shows that infertile women display significantly higher levels of stress than fertile women. So stress doesn't cause infertility, but infertility does cause stress.

Similarly, if your friend or family member offers up some nugget of advice about IVF that he read in last Sunday's health supplement, it is important to explain, again calmly, that you have read up extensively on the options available to you, have discussed these with your doctor or your support network, and are really doing everything you can already.

The best way to avoid such clashes is to educate those around you. The more they know about infertility, and about your problems (should you choose to tell them), the less they will upset you. The next section contains advice specifically for family and friends. If you would like more information to pass on to your family and friends, you can contact the National Infertility Support and Information Group (NISIG) online at *www.infertilityireland.ie* or on 1890 647 444.

3. Choose a private time to talk

Plan to talk to your friend or family member at a time when you know you will have their full attention. If one of you is in a hurry, or there are other people around, you may not be able to say everything you want to say, in the way you want to say it. It is also important to be somewhere where you can show as much emotion as you want, where you can feel free to cry if you need to.

4. Let your loved one know how to help you

It is a very good idea to decide how much, or how little, support and intervention you think you need, and to talk about it with your loved one. Most people with no prior experience of infertility don't really know what to say and do, and may welcome your advice.

Decide whether you want people to call you and ask you questions, or whether you would prefer to let them know when you have news to share. You will also need to decide whether or not you are going to share the dates of your treatment with family and friends. While it can be helpful to have support while you are going through investigations and procedures, it can be very stressful to have people asking about results. If you have a failed treatment cycle, you may wish to be left alone for some time to deal with your loss and to talk about what you want to do next. In that case, you may want to let some close family and friends know that you are having fertility treatment, but not let them in on the exact dates.

Your loved ones can also provide help and support by understanding that you will not always be up to attending certain family and social events. If you are at the end of a failed cycle or in the middle of a stressful one, or the event includes other people's pregnancies, babies or children, you will need to feel comfortable explaining that it will just be too hard for you to go.

5. Know when you've said enough

You will not always achieve a breakthrough by following the above advice. Sometimes your loved one will not understand, will not say the right thing. Sometimes they will challenge your carefully prepared words and try to tell you that you just need to do this or that. Sometimes they will be dismissive of your pain. You may find yourself battling for control of the conversation, and getting more and more upset at what you perceive to be their lack of understanding. If you do start to feel like it is a losing battle, the best thing you can do is to end the conversation, at least for the time being. All that will be gained by continuing to protest is that this person may end up thinking that the problem is not infertility, it is how you deal with it. And then they will tell you to relax.

Sometimes it is better to make a mental note not to discuss infertility with this person again. If it is very important to you that this person understands what you are going through, you need to go back to the drawing board and prepare again. Maybe their lack of understanding of the medical issues is the problem; perhaps they don't realise exactly what you have been through already. Again, education can be the key to the problem. You can contact your fertility clinic or NISIG for leaflets on infertility, or visit any of the websites listed in Chapter 4.

Louise from Dublin

Most of our family and friends didn't know we were doing IVF. Only my mum and a couple of close friends knew: they were very supportive and put up with me talking about it non-stop. It wasn't so much that it was a secret, but not everyone spreads the news when they're trying for a baby, and in essence this is what we were doing. We didn't want everyone hanging around for news about our IVF cycle.

When we were successful, and we told my husband's parents about the IVF, I was a bit surprised at their reaction. While they were delighted with the news, they wanted the IVF to be kept quiet and didn't want their relatives or neighbours and friends to know that the twins were 'test-tube babies'. I thought it was a bit old-fashioned, and felt a bit resentful, as I had no problems about it. I think, though, at the end of the day it's the 'generation gap': young people today are more in tune with the scientifics of their fertility and don't see anything wrong with it being helped along. It has tangled a bit of a web over the years: sometimes it's hard for me to remember who knows the twins are IVF, and who we're meant to churn out the 'Oh yes, there's twins in the family' story to!

Advice for family and friends

Most people know someone who is infertile. You may not know that they are, but with one in six couples seeking help to have a baby, there is a very good chance that a few of your family and friends are dealing with infertility. And yet there is little information available to friends and family who want to help.

Infertility is a very difficult and painful struggle. The research of Dr Alice Domar, professor at Harvard Medical School, suggests that the stress endured by infertility patients is comparable to that experienced by people undergoing treatment for cancer and AIDS.

The emotional pain of infertility can be likened to that of a loved one dying. However, when a loved one dies there is usually a period of grief and anger, eventually followed by acceptance, during which time you can begin to get on with your life.

For an infertile couple, this pain is recurring and continues to rear its ugly head month after month, year after year, with no let-up for a period of healing or acceptance. Every time a cycle fails, the couple must simply endure the loss of the baby they will not get to hold in eight months. No matter how many cycles have failed in the past, each month they get their hopes up and plan their future, only to be knocked down and kicked in the guts yet again. It is like having a loved one on life support, with the promise every month that they might come round.

Life gets even harder when the couple starts fertility treatment. In Ireland, fertility treatment is very expensive and is not covered by any medical insurers. The hormones involved can also be very hard on the woman's body; this only adds to the levels of stress experienced by the couple. The failure of a fertility-treatment cycle can take several months and even longer for a couple to come to terms with.

So how can you help?

There is no one way in which you can help your loved one deal with the pain of infertility. That is because different people deal with the strain in different ways, and also because the stress and emotions a couple goes through can vary depending on what stage of the journey they are at. Nevertheless, there are certain dos and don'ts that will help bring you closer to the friend or family member who is suffering infertility, and hopefully help you go some way towards helping them.

1. Listen and learn

Listen carefully to everything your loved one tells you about their infertility journey. Trust that what they tell you is the truth and that their feelings are valid. Don't say 'You can't possibly feel that bad' or 'You don't really mean that'. If your loved one tells you that the pain of infertility is worse than the pain they felt when they lost a parent, then you have to accept that this is true.

Pay attention if your loved one wants to discuss any investigations or treatment that they are having. If they are telling you, then it is important to them that you know and understand what is going on. And the more you know about what they are going through, the more you can help make things easier for them.

2. Avoid platitudes

The most important piece of advice I can give you is that it is better to say nothing at all than to say the wrong thing. You may not know what to say and feel like offering words of consolation such as 'I just know it will happen for you soon'. Unless you can provide your loved one with a bona fide guarantee that it will indeed happen soon (which of course you cannot), these words will mean nothing to them and may even upset them. If you feel awkward and don't know what to say, then the best thing you can say is 'Sorry', and give the person a hug.

Don't say 'It could be worse'. You don't know that it could be. If having a child is all the couple has ever dreamed of, maybe it couldn't be worse.

Don't say 'Maybe you're not meant to have children'. You wouldn't say to a short-sighted person 'Maybe you're not meant to see further than your nose'. Infertility is a medical condition, and thankfully one that can be successfully treated in the majority of cases.

3. Don't offer unsolicited advice

By the time an infertile couple has decided to look for help, they probably already know more about trying to conceive than any fertile couple has ever needed to know. They will know all about timed intercourse, ovulation, fertility signs; they will have sought advice from magazines, books and websites about diet, vitamins and supplements. It is also likely that they have looked into possible problems that might be preventing them from having a baby. Once they have started medical investigations, they will have talked through their treatment options with their doctor and will be as informed as they need to be.

Don't say to your loved one: 'Have you thought about IVF?' That is like saying to a cancer patient: 'Have you thought about chemotherapy?' If it is the right option for the couple, then they will have thought long and hard about it and will have discussed it with their doctor. If it is not for them, they will also have discussed it and ruled it out, or postponed it for a later date if necessary. If you have read an article on fertility treatment, don't present your findings as new information that is bound to help. If it is available in the mainstream media, the infertile couple has probably read up on it a long time ago.

Don't offer inspirational stories about your friend's aunt's cousin who did eight IVFs, had five miscarriages and eventually went on to have a baby. There are three things wrong with this story. Firstly, your friend's aunt's cousin has a baby (and good for her), but your loved one does not. Secondly, your friend's aunt's cousin having a baby is not going to help your loved one. And finally, telling your loved one that they may have to endure that much loss and pain along the way is not going to make them feel any better.

4. Educate yourself

One of the best things you can do to support your loved one is to read up as much as possible about what they are going through. That way, you can talk to them on their level about the investigations they are having done, or the treatments they are enduring. Not only will this help you avoid offering them platitudes and unsolicited advice, they will also appreciate that you care enough to do this.

5. If you're not sure, ask

If you don't know how to act or what to say, ask your loved one. Only they can tell you the best thing to do. It may be that they find things too hard to talk about at the moment – in which case you need to accept that they want some privacy or solitude. Be prepared for this response, as there will be times like these.

The rest of the time, they will appreciate that you are looking for guidance instead of trying to push guidance upon them – something that well-meaning but ill-informed friends of infertiles tend to do a lot. This piece of advice is most important if you are pregnant or have children yourself.

Val from Waterford

As a couple who have been diagnosed with 'unexplained infertility', we have nothing we can point the finger at and 'blame' for our inability to conceive. As such, fielding questions from well-meaning family and friends can be a minefield.

When a person who isn't aware of our journey through infertility asks a seemingly innocent and friendly question (such as 'You two have been married a few years now, any pitter-patter of tiny feet to be heard yet?'), it can be hard to know how to react. Do you brush it off with a laugh and pretend you haven't even thought about having children yet, and sure, maybe at some stage in the future you will, or do you take a more serious tack, and gently remind them that it's not always a case of just 'deciding' to have children for some couples. Of course then you have perhaps opened yourself up to a multitude of questions, if the person realises that you are one of those couples; you might not want everyone knowing the personal details and heartaches of your life.

Sometimes it's all you can do to smile and reply 'not yet', all the time trying to hold back the tears at the unexpected reminder of the absence of that baby you've been longing for for years and had assumed would just show up, bang on schedule, when you decided as a couple you were ready to have children.

It's a completely different matter, however, when family and friends are aware of your situation. Their approach can vary from being overly cautious – to the point of avoiding so much as mentioning children or babies, so as not to upset you – to being overly involved, with daily questions from well-meaning people who are

---

177

hoping and praying you will finally 'hit the jackpot' after such a long time trying. Sometimes the well-meaning can come to you with information, assuming that they're doing you a favour, and perhaps not realising that you have probably already encountered almost everything there is to know about infertility on your own journey.

Either approach can at times be upsetting, depending on how strong you are feeling, or indeed where you are in your treatment or your cycle. The overly involved serve to remind you daily of your 'failing', whereas the overly cautious may sometimes come across as uncaring and thoughtless. It's a tricky balancing act to pull off if you're a friend of someone who is experiencing problems. The best course of action is probably to take the cue from your friend, listening if he or she wants to talk. A simple 'How are you keeping?' every now and then might be enough to let them know you are thinking of them and are there if they want to talk.

Catherine from Cork

I have had the most supportive and wonderful friends – and also the most appalling lack of thought displayed by people who are not perhaps privy to our journey.

The good friends are ones who will at times ask you how you are coping, leaving it open to you whether you want to go into depth and have a shoulder to cry on, or if you want to just say 'Doing OK at the moment, thanks' and leave it at that. They will listen to you when you get yet another disappointment, and let you cry and rant at the world without passing judgement.

The worst experiences I have had in dealing with friends and family are mainly with people who are not aware of our problem in conceiving. I had the most appalling time while in work, as many of the other women in my office were announcing their pregnancies and intention of being out on maternity leave. That in itself was painful at times, but bearable. What was not bearable, however, was when people started rounding on me and asking what was taking so long: 'Sure you're married ages now, when are you going?'

The icing on the cake was when some of the women, in high spirits one day, started jesting with our boss that there might be another member of staff asking for leave soon, and doing the whole nudge-nudge wink-wink routine, pointing at me, implying that I might have 'some news'. I had to explain, red-faced, to our boss, that no, I was not in fact pregnant, the women were only having a little fun winding him up at the thoughts of another employee being absent for the guts of a year. That, of course, was then followed swiftly by a dash to the loos by me, so I could cry my eyes out because of my longing to be able to say those two simple words: 'I'm pregnant.'

I've had less-than-pleasant experiences upon telling some family members about our situation too. When I confided in one family member, her reaction was 'You're so lucky. Sure you're better off without children, isn't it great to think you never have to worry about getting pregnant accidentally now!' and she went off on a diatribe about how much time and money children cost. Well, I'd like to have the choice to be able to decide for myself if I want to get pregnant, thanks very much. I don't consider infertility a 'lucky' thing to suffer from.

I have personally found that you should pick and choose carefully whom you confide in. A few close friends or family members can help you through the tough times, and be a rock of support, but I have learned to keep my cards close to my chest with most people. While most people try their best to be supportive, sometimes that well-meaning support can be overwhelming and upsetting, as your moods and emotions continue on the merry-go-round of ups and downs on the seemingly endless cycle of infertility.

Looking after each other

Finally, don't forget to look after each other. This is a very difficult time for both of you, and while some people find it brings them closer together, other couples find that the stress can start to take its toll on a previously strong relationship.

There will be times when one of you is up and the other is down: try to be the supportive one when it is your turn. And when you are down, try to remember that being the supportive one can often be just as hard.

Take time out from infertility. Limit the time you talk about it in the evenings – allow yourselves twenty minutes, say, and then force yourselves to change the subject. Take a day trip or a weekend away, and promise each other that you will talk about other things.

Do the things that made you happy before you started TTC. This might sound like an empty piece of advice, but once TTC becomes the main driving force in your lives, it can be easy to forget about everything else you once enjoyed. Don't stop listening to music, going to gigs, reading books, going to the cinema or having a laugh with your friends. It may be hard to see it now, but there are more things in life than babies, and you don't have to put all those things on hold until your baby comes along.

Notes

1   Stanton, Annette L. et al, 'Psychosocial aspects of selected issues in women's reproductive health: Current status and future directions', *Journal of Consulting and Clinical Psychology*, June 2002, 70(3), 751–70

2   Anderheim L. et al, 'Does psychological stress affect the outcome of in vitro fertilization?', *Human Reproduction*, 2005, 20(10), 2969–75

3   Baik Seok Kee et al, 'A study on psychological strain in IVF patients', *Journal of Assisted Reproduction and Genetics*, 2000, 17(8), 461–85

9

Dealing with miscarriage

Introduction

When you lose a child, you lose your future. It doesn't matter how long your baby has been with you: you will feel the gap that their death has left behind. From the moment we know about our babies, we plan their future, *our* future, together. We work out our due dates, pick names, imagine who they will look like. When these hopes and dreams are taken away from us, it often seems like we are expected to forget we ever had them.

Dealing with the death of a baby is different to dealing with the death of a grandparent or a parent. Then there is a framework for dealing with grief, remembering the past and slowly moving forward to acceptance. When you lose a baby, acceptance can be very difficult. We want to know why it happened, if it was our fault, if there was anything we could have done to prevent it. And we want to know how we can prevent it happening again, and how we will deal with the fear of losing another baby, should we be lucky enough to get another chance.

When a couple has already dealt with infertility, pregnancy loss can seem like the cruellest blow. You may feel that nothing makes any sense any more, that if there was any justice in the world, your baby would not have died. Not only do we have to grieve for the baby we will never get to hold, we also have to face back into the dark depths of infertility if we wish to try again.

Sadly, we are not talking about a small minority of pregnancies here. Approximately one in four pregnancies will end before their time, most of those in the first twelve weeks. You may be surprised to read that miscarriage is so common. You may also be surprised by the number of people who may confess their own stories of pregnancy loss to you, once you have told them of yours. It is not something that was spoken of in our parents' time, and even now it is not dinner-party-discussion material.

However, it is important to acknowledge your little one's existence, to be able to talk through your grief with the people who care about you, and to remind those people that you had a baby that you loved and will always remember. Your loved ones may not always say or do the right thing, but try not to hold that against them. If they are prepared to listen, you can try to explain how you are feeling. There is no easy way of dealing with the grief, but talking, crying and venting are good ways to start. I have to be honest and say that the only thing that has helped me move on from miscarriage is another pregnancy, but we still have to live our lives to the best of our abilities, whether or not we will ever be fortunate enough to conceive again.

Type of loss

Early miscarriage
An early miscarriage is one that occurs before the thirteenth week of pregnancy. Most of these occur by eight weeks' gestation.

Late miscarriage
A miscarriage is considered late if it occurs after the thirteenth week of pregnancy. In Ireland, pregnancy loss between thirteen and twenty-four weeks is considered a miscarriage. A loss at this stage is fairly uncommon, and happens in less than 1 percent of pregnancies.

Stillbirth
In Ireland, stillbirth is the death of a baby after the twenty-fourth week of pregnancy, but prior to delivery. When a baby lives for only a short time after birth, his or her death is referred to as a neonatal death.

Biochemical pregnancy
A biochemical pregnancy is one that occurs when the embryo does not implant properly in the uterine lining, and so the pregnancy cannot continue. When the embryo begins to implant, it will start to produce HCG, so the pregnancy is capable of being detected on a home pregnancy test. When implantation starts to fail, the lines will become fainter or disappear completely, and your period will begin soon afterwards.

Anembryonic miscarriage

An anembryonic miscarriage, also known as a blighted ovum, happens when the fertilised egg implants into the uterine lining but then fails to develop. There is usually a pregnancy sac containing placental tissue but no embryo. Recent research suggests that the empty sac once contained an embryo but that the embryo was reabsorbed early in its development. Anembryonic miscarriages are among the most common types of early miscarriage.

Embryonic miscarriage

An embryonic miscarriage is the name given to a miscarriage that occurs after a foetal heartbeat has developed. It is important to differentiate between an anembryonic and an embryonic miscarriage, as the underlying cause may be different.

Complete miscarriage

A miscarriage is said to be complete when all the products of conception, including the foetus and the placental tissue, are expelled from the uterus. The symptoms are heavy bleeding and the passing of blood clots and tissue. If you are worried that any tissue has been left behind, an ultrasound will be able to detect whether this is the case.

Incomplete miscarriage

Sometimes not all of the products of conception are passed from the uterus, and the miscarriage is deemed to be incomplete. An ultrasound can show if there is any remaining tissue; this usually consists of pieces of placenta and membranes from the pregnancy sac. These can be removed under anaesthetic during a D&C (dilation and curettage) or an ERPC (evacuation of retained products of conception). These are routine procedures that take about twenty minutes.

Missed miscarriage

A missed miscarriage occurs when the foetus or embryo dies in the uterus and, instead of being expelled, is retained. There may be some light bleeding or cramping, or pregnancy symptoms may ease, but frequently there is no indication that anything is wrong. Often, a missed miscarriage is only detected when no heartbeat can be found at a routine ultrasound, and the foetus or embryo is smaller than it should be. If no action is taken, the uterus will usually expel the pregnancy in time. However, many women prefer to have a D&C or ERPC in order to help their physical and emotional recovery.

Ectopic pregnancy

An ectopic pregnancy occurs when the fertilised egg implants outside of the uterus. This usually happens in the fallopian tubes but may also happen on the ovary or in the abdominal cavity. An ectopic pregnancy is never viable, as there is not enough room for the embryo to grow, or for the placenta to implant properly. Sometimes an ectopic pregnancy will miscarry without complication, but if it continues to grow, it can cause severe pain and even rupture the walls of the fallopian tube, resulting in the loss of the tube.

The first sign of an ectopic pregnancy is lower-abdominal pain, which is usually followed by bleeding. If you experience this combination of symptoms, you should contact your doctor immediately. An ultrasound will be able to tell whether there is a pregnancy sac in the uterus, although it may be difficult to see whether there is a sac or a foetal heartbeat outside of the uterus. If there is any doubt about the diagnosis, the doctor may perform a laparoscopy. The ectopic can then either be removed by surgery, or an injection of methotrexate can be administered. This stops the pregnancy from developing, and the sac will eventually shrivel away. HCG levels should be monitored to ensure that the pregnancy has ended.

Molar pregnancy

A hydatidiform mole is a growth that forms inside the uterus, at the beginning of a pregnancy, instead of a foetus. It is usually an overgrowth of placental tissue, which resembles a bunch of grapes, as the placental cells are swollen with fluid. These moles can be complete or partial. Partial moles are much more common and usually mimic the appearance of an incomplete miscarriage. Often, the diagnosis is only made after the tissue has been removed by an ERPC. In a small number of cases, complete moles can develop into an invasive cancer, so specialist follow-up treatment is needed.

Recurrent miscarriage

In Ireland, recurrent miscarriage is diagnosed after three or more consecutive miscarriages. It is uncommon, affecting about 1 percent of women. Recurrent miscarriage can be due to bad luck, but it is also possible that there is an underlying cause. After three consecutive miscarriages, most doctors will recommend investigations in order to find, or at least rule out, certain conditions.

Miscarriage causes, investigations and treatments

One of your first questions is likely to be: why did this happen? Unfortunately, in most cases, the cause of miscarriage will not be determined. Many doctors and clinics will not conduct investigations until a third consecutive miscarriage. This can be a very frustrating and upsetting policy for those couples who have suffered a second miscarriage and want to do everything in their power to ensure that they do not have to endure a third. However, most studies have found that most women who have suffered one or two consecutive miscarriages will indeed go on to carry to term on a subsequent pregnancy and will not join the ranks of the recurrent miscarriers. The factors that cause sporadic, or once-off, miscarriages are usually different from the factors that cause recurrent miscarriage, and thus sporadic miscarriage is unlikely to be repeated.

Because of this, it is simply not efficient for public hospitals to investigate the cause of every miscarriage, and most couples will just be told to go off and try again. If you are attending a private obstetrician or gynaecologist, he or she may be prepared to conduct some tests for you, should you wish.

Even if investigations are conducted, a cause may not be found. No reason was ever found for my six miscarriages, despite extensive testing. Just bad luck? Unlikely, but possible.

Chromosomal abnormalities

A chromosomal abnormality in the embryo is the most common cause of miscarriage. The chromosomal defect can occur before, during or after the process of fertilisation and can cause an abnormal embryo to develop. The vast majority of chromosomal abnormalities are incompatible with life, and the woman's body will reject the embryo early in the pregnancy. This is the cause of more than 50 percent of early miscarriages. There are many types of chromosomal abnormality but the most common defects are trisomies (where the cells contain three copies of one type of chromosome instead of the usual two), monosomies (where one of the chromosomes is completely missing) and polyploids (where the embryo contains one or more extra sets of twenty-three chromosomes). In most cases, these chromosomal anomalies are random and are unlikely to occur again. However, as a woman ages, the likelihood of her eggs containing abnormalities increases.

Although most chromosomal abnormalities are unlikely to reoccur, it is possible that an abnormality in one of the parent's chromosomes may be the cause of recurrent miscarriage. The most common of these abnormalities is a balanced translocation, where a fragment of one chromosome becomes attached to the broken end of another. It is 'balanced' because the abnormality affects only one of the chromosome pairs; as a result, the parent with the translocation appears to be entirely normal.

If you have suffered recurrent miscarriage, your doctor may suggest that you both have a blood test to check for chromosomal problems. This test is referred to as karyotyping. About 5 percent of couples who suffer recurrent miscarriage will have this problem. If either of you has a chromosomal abnormality, you will be referred to a genetic counsellor (if you are not referred automatically, you should ask for a referral), who will advise you of your risks and options.

Infections

Certain bacterial infections are known to have the potential to cause miscarriage. However, they are a rare cause of recurrent miscarriage, as most are detectable and treatable.

Syphilis is known to cause miscarriage. All pregnant women in Ireland are tested for this disease, and it is easily treated with antibiotics, so it is now a rare cause of miscarriage. Herpes is also a known cause of miscarriage, although the foetus is only infected during the mother's first herpes infection, even though the mother may experience repeat episodes herself.

Rubella, listeriosis and toxoplasmosis can all cause miscarriage (although this, again, is rare), so a simple pre-pregnancy blood test is recommended to rule out these infections. Also, if rubella antibodies are not present, a vaccination is recommended before you start TTC.

Bacterial vaginosis, an infection that causes the vaginal secretions to be more alkaline than usual, has recently been recognised as a cause of late miscarriage. This condition can be diagnosed using a cervical smear. Some studies have also suggested that it could be a cause of early miscarriage. Bacterial vaginosis can be treated with antibiotics, although this may not prevent the infection causing preterm labour.

Any infection that causes a very high temperature runs the risk of affecting the foetus and, in extreme cases, causing miscarriage. If you have a high temperature while pregnant, you should seek medical help immediately.

Hormonal causes

The menstrual cycle is a delicately balanced process (see Chapter 2) that can be disrupted by many different factors. In some cases, an imbalance in hormones will result in an inability to conceive. In other cases, conception may occur but there may not be an adequate supply of the appropriate hormones to sustain the pregnancy.

Low progesterone is often cited as a cause of miscarriage. If the corpus luteum does not produce an adequate amount of progesterone or it does not produce it for a long enough period, the embryo may fail to implant properly and die. A simple blood test can check your progesterone level at seven days after ovulation to see if it is at an adequate level. If it is low, many doctors prescribe progesterone supplements in the hope that this will help sustain a pregnancy, but others feel that the low progesterone is a symptom rather than a cause of miscarriage and that supplementation does little more than sustain a pregnancy that is already failing. Progesterone supplements do no harm (except perhaps by prolonging a non-viable pregnancy) and can provide reassurance to women, so many doctors who are unconvinced by their effectiveness will prescribe them for patients.

Another way of helping progesterone production is to improve the overall quality of ovulation from the start, so that a better-quality, or better-matured, egg will result in a better corpus luteum. One way of doing this is to use the fertility drug Clomid (see Chapter 7) early in the menstrual cycle. Other fertility drugs (see Chapter 7) may also be prescribed for this purpose.

HCG (human chorionic gonadotropin, the pregnancy hormone) shots may also be prescribed to try to sustain a pregnancy. HCG is produced by the embryo once it implants in the uterine lining, and its production sends a feedback message to the corpus luteum to keep producing progesterone. However, there is no evidence that HCG shots help prevent miscarriage. Again, some doctors prescribe them anyway, as they can provide reassurance to women who have suffered a previous miscarriage, and they do no harm.

Hormonal problems that result from diabetes or an under- or overactive thyroid have been suggested as causes of miscarriage. However, it is extremely unlikely that a woman with diabetes or a thyroid problem will first present with symptoms following a miscarriage. In fact, both problems are much more likely to be diagnosed and treated as a cause of infertility, or as problems in their own right. Once they have been diagnosed and treated, they are very unlikely to be a cause of miscarriage.

Autoimmune disorders

Autoimmune disorders occur when the immune system produces antibodies that attack and destroy healthy body tissue. The auto-antibodies that are most strongly associated with miscarriage are the antiphospholipid family of antibodies (APA). These antibodies can cause clotting in the blood vessels of the placenta, which can stop the placenta working properly; this can in turn lead to the death of the baby. Unfortunately, many women with APA will not find out about this condition until they are undergoing investigations for recurrent miscarriage. A blood test can check for the main types of APA, which are lupus anticoagulant and anticardiolipin antibodies. About one in six recurrent miscarriers has the APA syndrome.

The most effective treatment for women with APA is the use of aspirin and heparin. Aspirin, which is taken in tablet form, and heparin, which is injected, both thin the blood and improve the blood flow through the placenta.

Abnormalities of the uterus and cervix

There are a number of congenital uterine abnormalities that are associated with infertility and miscarriage (more on these in Chapter 6). The most highly associated with miscarriage is the septate uterus, whereby the inside of the uterus is divided by a wall, or septum. The septum may extend part of the way into the uterus, or can reach as far as the cervix. The septum has no blood flow, and this can interfere with implantation and cause miscarriage. A bicornuate uterus, which is heart-shaped, with a deep indentation at the top, is associated with late miscarriage and preterm labour, as there is often not enough room for the baby to grow to term.

Some uterine abnormalities can be diagnosed with a simple ultrasound: for instance, a bicornuate uterus can often be seen clearly. However, even if a uterine abnormality can be identified using ultrasound, a hysteroscopy or laparoscopy (see Chapter 6), or both, is usually used for a full diagnosis. Treatment can then be carried out also by hysteroscopy or laparoscopy, either at the time of diagnosis or at a future date.

Uterine fibroids are benign growths that develop within the lining of the uterus. They can grow on their own or in clusters and can vary in size from a few millimetres to about 20 centimetres. If the fibroids are submucous (which means they push into the uterine cavity), they can cause miscarriage. Uterine fibroids can be removed by a procedure known as a myomectomy (see Chapter 6). Intrauterine adhesions and endometrial polyps (see Chapter 6) have also been associated with miscarriage but are more likely to be the cause of infertility.

Cervical incompetence can be a cause of late miscarriage, preterm labour and stillbirth. This happens when the cervix opens before the baby has developed to a size where it can live outside the uterus. Unfortunately, this is not usually diagnosed until the cervix has opened unexpectedly during pregnancy. If a woman has suffered a loss due to cervical incompetence in a previous pregnancy, a stitch can be inserted into the cervix on a subsequent pregnancy, to stop it dilating.

Physical management of miscarriage

Your medical practitioner may advise a specific method for the management of your miscarriage. Surgical removal (a D&C) has been the method of choice in the past fifty years, as doctors believed that leaving retained tissue in the uterus could cause dangerous bleeding. Current obstetrical practice has moved away from surgical removal as a matter of course, as many obstetricians believe that a woman's body is capable of passing the tissue on its own, and so an invasive surgical procedure, with its associated risks, is not necessarily done.

There is also the option of taking drugs to speed up the process. A prostaglandin can be administered to encourage the uterus to contract and expel its contents. For some women, this may be preferable to undergoing surgery and a general anaesthetic, but this should be weighed up against the physical and emotional trauma of contractions and the subsequent passing of the pregnancy sac and the foetus.

The stage at which the miscarriage has occurred is also an important consideration when deciding on how to proceed. If a pregnancy is lost before six weeks, there is probably no need for a surgical procedure, as there is only a small amount of tissue to be passed. If your miscarriage has occurred between six and eight weeks, your medical practitioner may advise you on your choices. Unless there is evidence to the contrary, it will probably be safe for you to have a natural miscarriage, if that is what you choose. However, if you wish to have the tissue tested to try to understand the reason for the miscarriage, a D&C is advisable at any stage.

Between eight and twelve weeks of pregnancy, or if you have had a missed miscarriage, you will probably be advised to have a D&C, although there is still a possibility of a natural miscarriage. You will need to seek advice from your doctor about this.

When a baby is sixteen weeks or more, your doctors will probably advise you that you will need to be induced in order to go into labour, so that you can deliver the baby vaginally. A prostaglandin pessary is inserted into the vagina to start contractions. This may sound very frightening, but rest assured that your medical team will have access to all the pain relief that you might need.

D&C versus natural miscarriage

Whether you opt for a natural miscarriage or a surgical removal is a very personal decision. Most couples are bewildered when faced with the news that their baby has died, and are not necessarily in a position to make an informed decision on how to pass their baby, especially if it is their first miscarriage.

If you were less than six weeks pregnant and have already started to miscarry, it might be easier to allow the miscarriage process to continue naturally. You will bleed heavily for at least a week and will pass clots and tissue; this may be preferable to the stress of having to go to hospital, however.

If you were more than six weeks pregnant, and your medical practitioner is happy for you to miscarry naturally, you need to weigh up the stress of having an invasive procedure versus the trauma of passing your baby on your own. Some women would prefer to avoid a surgical procedure at all costs, and thankfully a natural miscarriage can be managed safely in many circumstances. However, you should be aware that a natural miscarriage can be very painful. You will bleed heavily, possibly for several weeks, you will pass large clots, and you may even be able to identify the pregnancy sac and the foetus. If you have had a missed miscarriage, then you will also have to wait for the process to begin, which can also be very traumatic.

A D&C can speed up both the miscarriage process and the recovery process. It also avoids the patient having to witness the passing of the pregnancy sac, tissue and foetus, as all tissue is removed during the twenty-minute procedure. You may bleed for a week or so afterwards and spot for another week or so after that.

If you wish to have tests done, it is preferable to have a D&C, as the tissue from a natural miscarriage is far more difficult to use for chromosomal testing, or to understand if a woman's immune system contributed to the death of a genetically viable baby. This is because by the time the tissue has been passed, there will have been extensive changes in the body to protect the woman from bleeding excessively during the process.

In my own personal experience, I found the recovery after a D&C at twelve weeks easier than passing the baby naturally at five and a half weeks. The bleeding was lighter, the cramping was milder, and I didn't have to witness the passing of clots and large amounts of tissue every time I went to the toilet. In both cases, my period returned exactly four weeks later.

Derval from Dublin

One afternoon, eleven weeks into my pregnancy, I started bleeding. It was light and brown: nothing to worry about, my GP told me. But by the next morning, things had got worse, so I went to hospital.

The doctor gave me an internal scan. There was a pregnancy sac but no heartbeat, no baby. It seemed the baby hadn't developed at all, or had died several weeks before and had been re-absorbed. She gave me the option of having a D&C while I was there or going home and waiting it out. I was incredibly upset and terrified at the idea of a general anaesthetic, so I went home. I tried to sleep but could only cry. After a while, the cramps became stronger, as painful as early-labour contractions, and the bleeding got heavier. I started passing large clots. It was horrendous, my body was expelling all that was there to nourish my baby. The worst part, and something that will always stay with me, was passing the foetal sac and seeing the little shrivelled pouch where my baby should have been.

By that evening, I could take no more and rang the hospital. I didn't know who I should talk to and, in tears, explained the situation to several nurses and receptionists before I got to speak to the right person. I was told it was too late to have the procedure done that day but that I could come in and spend the night in hospital. I just wanted it to be over, and if it couldn't be over, I thought I might as well stay at home. Thankfully, within a few hours the cramping eased somewhat.

After a week, I went back to the hospital for a follow-up appointment. The scan revealed everything was back to 'normal': my body had done a brutally efficient job. I still regret that I didn't have the D&C; losing my baby was bad enough, but the reality of physically losing her was truly harrowing, and I still get flashes of it now, two years later.

Dealing with your baby's remains

Early miscarriage

No matter how old your baby was, your hospital will be able to help you decide what to do with the baby's remains. The hospital chaplain is usually the person to talk to about this, and he or she can advise you.

If you have had a natural miscarriage, you have probably not held on to any of the baby's tissue. It can be extremely distressing for the couple to do this; however, some choose to do so, either so that the tissue can be tested, or so that it can be buried. If you wish to have the tissue tested, you can talk to your obstetrician; if you wish to bury your baby's remains, then you should talk to the hospital chaplain.

If you have had a D&C, you can talk to your obstetrician about having the tissue tested, should you wish to do so. Many hospitals will only do this once a woman has experienced three consecutive miscarriages. However, anecdotal evidence suggests that it is possible to overcome this obstacle: many women who have pushed for testing have managed to get it done after two, and sometimes just one, miscarriage. I did not experience any resistance when I asked for tests after my second miscarriage.

Before your D&C, the hospital chaplain may talk to you about your baby's remains. If you do not wish to deal with this yourself, your hospital team can do it for you. If you wish to bury your baby, the chaplain can organise this for you. If you do not get an opportunity to talk to the chaplain before your D&C, then make sure that your obstetrician is aware that you wish to bury your baby's remains.

Late miscarriage

If your miscarriage has happened at sixteen weeks or later, you will probably be induced to give birth to your baby. Delivering your baby, knowing that you won't get to bring him or her home, is a heartbreaking ordeal. You will probably be asked if you wish to see your baby. Most women find that it helps with the healing process to have memories of their baby. Many take photographs and footprints of their baby as keepsakes. One woman, who has endured two late miscarriages, confessed that she experienced regret that she had not seen and held her first son, whereas she cherished the time she spent with her second. Another woman says that she almost didn't have the courage to hold her baby, but changed her mind at the last minute, and is extremely thankful that she got to hold her daughter.

If you choose not to see your baby, the hospital can organise for a photo to be taken. This can either be given to you or kept with your hospital notes in case you would like to see it at a later date.

Your doctors may suggest that your baby undergoes a post-mortem examination to try to identify a cause of death. During the post-mortem, small amounts of tissue are taken from the baby's body. Once this has been done done, the body is repaired so that you can see and hold your baby again, should you wish.

You can talk to the hospital chaplain about how you wish to proceed once your baby's body is ready to leave the hospital. If you wish to bury or cremate your baby, the chaplain can organise the necessary paperwork and procedures, and help with funeral and burial arrangements.

Amy from Dublin

I was exactly nineteen weeks when I had my routine check-up with my GP. The first thing I asked her to do was to listen to baby's heartbeat. I had been nervous throughout the pregnancy as I'd lost my baby's twin at eight and a half weeks. As I lay on the bed and she tried to get the heartbeat, I began to realise that she was getting worried. After ten minutes – which seemed like a lifetime to me – she decided to call the hospital and advised me to go for a scan immediately.

I and my husband arrived at the hospital and went straight to the emergency area. As we waited for someone to come and scan us, we were both feeling sick. A midwife scanned us but said that she couldn't get a good picture. Then two more midwives arrived and scanned in silence for a few minutes before eventually saying that things didn't look good. They couldn't really differentiate between the baby and the placenta, and there was no heartbeat. We had lost our baby.

There was a lot of crying, but mostly there was shock. I couldn't believe that this could be happening to us, at nineteen weeks. It just wasn't fair. We were taken to see the doctor, who informed me that because I was over twelve weeks, I would have to give birth. I asked was there no other way, and he said no. I didn't think I could do it. He gave me tablets to take and told me to come back in two days. I wanted to know what our baby would look like. He said it was a very small baby but they couldn't be sure how complete he would be.

For two days I cried and cried and felt so numb. I tried to think of answers: why, why us, why me, why our baby? I was really concerned about what he would look like. I was frightened that he mightn't really look like a baby, and that would be awful for us.

Our baby came very quickly and easily in the end. I was lucky in that way. A lot of women have a tough time. Although we had thought a lot about what his appearance would be like, the only thing that took us a little by surprise was his colour: he was a very dark reddish colour, as he was only nineteen weeks. The midwife asked my husband if he'd like to cut the cord, which he did. It was the proudest yet saddest moment of my life, and one we'll never forget. The midwife, who was a lovely person and treated our baby and us with great respect, took our baby away to clean him up. She then brought our baby back in a tiny white box with a tiny blue sheet over him, and asked us if we'd like to name him, which we did. From then on, she referred to our baby by his name, which made us feel like he really was a person. She gave him to us to hold him and then left us alone.

We really looked closely at him then. Amazingly, he looked perfect: tiny enough to fit in my hand, but perfectly formed. We could even see his tongue, his hands and feet were tiny but perfect, and there were even tiny nail beds on his fingers and toes. We were scared at first to touch him, but after a few minutes we really felt that he was our son, and the love we had for him came out. Although we were devastated, these moments will be held in our hearts forever.

Finally, we said goodbye to our baby and left the hospital. I felt terribly guilty for leaving him, especially as it was the last time we'd see him properly. We'd decided to allow the hospital to perform a post-mortem, and it was explained to us that we wouldn't see our baby as he was again: when we'd get him back, he'd be covered in bandages. They said it could be up to six weeks before his body was released to us for burial. I'll never forget that night when I got home, sitting on the couch. I just felt so, so numb. I was no longer pregnant. My baby was gone.

Saying goodbye to your baby

It doesn't matter how small your baby was, you can say goodbye in whatever way you choose. You should speak to the hospital chaplain and let him or her know exactly what your wishes are. If you are unsure what to do, the chaplain will be able to provide you with information on your options and help you come to a decision. Most maternity hospitals have their own graveyards, and your baby can either be buried here or in a graveyard of your choice.

There is also a communal plot in Glasnevin Cemetery in Dublin for babies who have been the victims of miscarriage, stillbirth and neonatal death. This is called the Holy Angels plot. There are several rows of graves, with about sixteen babies buried in each grave. There is an individual headstone for each grave, with each baby's name engraved on it. The graves are decorated with flowers and toys; it is a wonderful, colourful sight to behold. We buried one of our babies here and, as well as it being a great comfort to have a place to visit, it is also somewhere that our son loves to visit.

There are a number of costs and procedures associated with a burial; your hospital should be able to advise you on these. If your baby died before twenty-four weeks, you will need to get a letter from your hospital stating why your baby does not have a PPS number. If either of you pay PRSI, you should be eligible for a bereavement grant, which can be put towards the cost of the burial. You can find more information on this at *www.welfare.ie.*

Coping with the emotional trauma

Everyone deals with miscarriage differently, just as everyone deals with any death differently. There is no 'correct' method, no standard grieving period. It doesn't matter how or when the pregnancy ended, it will come as a huge shock, and you will experience overwhelming feelings of grief, anger and despair. This is entirely normal.

Allow yourself time to deal with your emotions. Don't try to pull yourself together, to get on with things. Take as much time off work as you need. If you would rather not tell your employers about your miscarriage, explain the situation to your obstetrician or GP, and they should write a suitable letter to allow you to take time off work.

After my first miscarriage, I found myself back in work three days later. I was still bleeding heavily, and was dazed and confused. I thought it would be better to get back to 'normal' as soon as possible. I was wrong. There is no 'normal' for a long time after miscarriage; sometimes it can change your perspective forever. After my second miscarriage, my obstetrician gave me a sick note for five weeks. I went on holiday for two weeks with my husband and son. Much better idea.

However, it may well be the best thing for you to get back to work and into a familiar routine. Only you can decide how you think you will cope best. As I said, there is no right or wrong thing to do.

Mourning your baby

Whether you are used to crying freely or would rather keep a tight rein on your emotions, you should allow yourself to cry as much as you feel you need to. I generally feel a little bit better after a good cry – if only until the next one – and it is good to get that feeling of reprieve.

Most people also find that it helps them to talk about their baby, to acknowledge its existence and the importance of its short life. I guarantee you that if you are prepared to open yourself up to people and talk about your baby, you will be surprised by how many people will admit to having experienced a loss too. Sadly, it is still something that is rarely discussed, and because of this, many of those around you may find it difficult and embarrassing to talk about your loss, and will struggle to find the right words. If you want to talk to them, you can let them know that all they need to do is listen, and that that in itself is a great help.

You may prefer to seek out like-minded people with whom to share your grief, as they are the only ones who will truly understand what you are going through. The Irish websites *www.rollercoaster.ie* and *www.magicmum.com* both have sections covering pregnancy loss, where you will receive support from those who have experienced losses. There is also plenty of advice for all aspects of pregnancy loss, and for trying again. You can find similar sections on most of the TTC websites mentioned in Chapter 4.

If you would prefer to talk to someone directly, or to meet others who have experienced a miscarriage, you can contact the Miscarriage Association of Ireland at *www.miscarriage.ie*. They have a telephone support line (this changes on a monthly basis depending on which member is providing the support) and organise monthly support meetings.

Men and miscarriage

As all the medical focus in relation to miscarriage is on the woman, it can be easy to forget that her partner has also lost his child. As a man, you may feel that it is your role to support your partner, look after her, and make sure all her needs are being met. It is also important to allow yourself the same luxuries. Take time off work, give yourself time to grieve, cry together, and spend time together doing things that make you both happy.

Each of you may react differently to the death of your baby. As I said before, there is no right or wrong way to behave or to grieve; everyone does it in their own way, and in their own time.

No matter how you both cope with the aftermath of the miscarriage, it is likely that your partner will be more deeply affected should you decide to try again. Many women find themselves desperate to be pregnant again, and feel that this is the only thing that can help them get over the loss of their baby. When a woman is that eager for another pregnancy, every failed cycle can feel like another miscarriage.

You may be overwhelmed by the depth of emotions that your partner is experiencing, and may feel powerless to help. The best thing you can do in this situation is to talk, and of course listen. In my experience, it is talking that gets couples through these difficult times. While it is true that miscarriage and TTC can bring couples closer together, for many it can drive them apart if emotions are suppressed and resentment is allowed to build up. If you are able to talk your way through each stage of your recovery, you will be able to move on sooner rather than later.

Coping with other people's reactions

If you decide to share the news of your miscarriage with family and friends, you may get a variety of reactions. Some people will be very understanding, especially those who have experienced miscarriage themselves. However, many people, who have not been through a miscarriage, may feel awkward and will not know what to say. They may reach for a platitude in an attempt to say something rather than nothing; you need to prepare for this situation.

'It was probably for the best', 'There was obviously something wrong with the baby', 'You can always try again', 'It just wasn't meant to be' and 'At least you know you can get pregnant'; generally no harm is meant by any of these statements – in fact, quite the opposite. If you are able to take them in the manner in which they were intended, it might be best to smile sweetly and move on. However, some people can find such platitudes very hurtful and upsetting, regardless of the intention of the speaker. If you feel up to it, you can reply with a firm but honest statement, such as 'I loved and wanted *this* baby'.

Or you can torture yourself by coming up with smart answers to all the usual platitudes. This is not recommended, but some people (OK, me) just can't help themselves!

Because little is said about miscarriage, there is not a generally accepted consensus on how to comfort those who have lost a baby, or indeed on whether or not a couple may need comforting at all. So you may find that it makes people uncomfortable to talk about your baby, or to be told why a well-meaning platitude has upset you. However, let's not forget that one in four pregnancies ends in miscarriage: it is a very common occurrence, and something that people shouldn't be afraid to talk about. And the more you tell people, the more you will realise that you are not alone.

For those who are wondering how best to express their condolences to others who have experienced a miscarriage, I always find that a simple 'sorry' is enough. I also appreciate when people ask me about the baby.

Coping with special dates

You have probably known your baby's due date from the moment you were aware that he or she existed – possibly even from the moment you ovulated. When your baby is gone, this date looms in the distance, reminding you of the future that was taken from you. For those trying again, it may serve as a date by which you hope to be pregnant again. Whatever your circumstances, it is an important day, and one you may wish to mark.

It will be a big day for you, but try to remember that it is just a day, similar to the one before it and the one after it. Try not to let the build-up to the day fill you with dread; instead, plan something for the day that both of you can enjoy together. Try to mark the anniversary of your miscarriage in a similar way, so that you can celebrate the short life of your baby as much as you will mourn the fact that he or she is no longer with you.

You may find other days of celebration difficult: birthdays, Christmas, Mother's Day and Father's Day. The days when everyone else seems to be happy can be the ones that make you feel the saddest. Again, remember that it is just one day, and that it will be over by tomorrow. If you feel up to it, you can do something just for yourselves: spoil yourselves, so that you have at least some moments of happiness during the day.

Remembering your baby

Some couples will have a grave to visit and tend, and this can be a great source of comfort. Many of those who have had early losses or have chosen not to bury their baby will still wish to have a memorial of some sort. One idea is to plant a tree or bush in memory of your little one. Some people have told me that they have chosen a plant that flowers around the time of their baby's due date. Those who do not have access to gardens – or green fingers! – might choose an ornament or a painting as a memorial. After my second miscarriage, a friend sent me a figurine of a child holding a balloon with the message 'Hope' on it. Perfect.

Dealing with recurrent miscarriage

Pregnancy after miscarriage is a very scary place. Every ache, twinge, and trip to the bathroom can leave you in a state of terror. If you have suffered more than one miscarriage, these feelings can be amplified, to the point where it's hard to relax at all. Then, when your worst fears are realised, the shock can be even more overwhelming than if you'd never anticipated it in the first place.

Recurrent miscarriage affects about 1 percent of couples. The term usually refers to those who have had three or more consecutive miscarriages. Despite the extensive testing available to help find an underlying cause for recurrent miscarriage, in about 50 percent of cases no cause is ever found. This can be extremely distressing for a couple who have no reason to believe that the next pregnancy will be any different from those that have gone before. However, recent research suggests that couples who experience up to five consecutive miscarriages still have a 60 percent chance of carrying a baby to term. It is only after more than five consecutive miscarriages that the chance of success starts to drop off.

One, two and sometimes even three consecutive miscarriages can be down to bad luck. However, it is advisable to have as many tests as possible done after three consecutive miscarriages (and after two, if you wish), in order to rule out any possible underlying causes, and to put your mind at rest.

While the physical side of recurrent miscarriage can become easier to deal with, as you have been through it before and know what to expect, the emotional side can be unbearable. You may constantly think 'Why?' and 'Why me?' as others seem to take a carefree pregnancy for granted. Feelings of anger, rage and jealousy are common, and you should not feel guilty about feeling the way you do. Try to find someone to talk to about how you are feeling: this can be your husband, a friend, a counsellor or members of a support group. The more people you talk to, the more you will realise that you have the support of others, and that you are not alone. A good starting point may be to find a recurrent-miscarriage support group online so that you can discuss your feelings with other people who have been through the same thing as you. *www.rollercoaster.ie* has a good Pregnancy Loss board with sections for those who have suffered from recurrent miscarriage.

Dealing with pregnancy loss and infertility

Miscarriage is a devastating blow for any couple, but if you have had serious problems conceiving, it can seem like the world has ended. You may feel as though you have paid your dues with infertility, and the loss of the baby you have wanted for so long seems impossible to come to terms with.

Many people will tell you that 'At least you know you can get pregnant' or that 'You can always try again', but those people may have little idea what 'trying again' means. Whether you have suffered endless months of disappointment before seeing those two lines, or have endured one painful and expensive fertility treatment after another, thinking about trying again may prove to be as difficult as coming to terms with your baby's death.

I remember lying on the scan bed wailing after my second miscarriage had been confirmed; the nurse tried to console me with kind words about my baby. I had to tell her that, while the death of my baby was extremely traumatic, it was the thought of returning to infertility that was causing most of my tears. It was the same in the hospital where I had my ERPC: the staff kept telling me that I could try again, that I would have a baby before long. Again, I had to explain that it wasn't that simple, and that we might never have a baby. They were used to dealing with miscarriage but were not so familiar with infertility.

If you come into contact with medical staff who are either unaware of your circumstances or are unsympathetic towards them, try to explain calmly and firmly why this is so difficult for you. Your hospital visit will be distressing enough, without having to listen to painful comments over and over again.

You may feel anger, despair and jealousy, not to mention deep sadness. It is very difficult to bear, but please believe me, it does get easier in time: you won't always feel this bad. It is helpful to talk to each other and to those who understand what you are going through. Many couples find counselling helpful at this point, both to help them deal with their loss and to help them move on to the next step. Both the National Infertility Support & Information Group (NISIG – *www.infertilityireland.ie*) and the Miscarriage Association of Ireland (*www.miscarriage.ie*) can help you find someone to talk to, and they also organise support groups. Your fertility clinic should also have a counsellor available to you.

Even if this is your first miscarriage, you may want to talk to your fertility clinic about tests you can have done to try to determine a cause of your baby's death. This is not done in the maternity hospitals after one miscarriage, but as you have had problems conceiving, there may be some related problems that have not been addressed. Cruel and unfair as it may seem, unfortunately miscarriage is more common amongst infertile couples.

Taking the next step is not easy. If you conceived naturally, you may be eager to try again as soon as possible, even if you are daunted by the prospect of another long haul. Or you may feel that you need some more time to come to terms with your loss. However, if you have had to pay for fertility treatments, being emotionally ready may not be enough. It is heartbreaking to think of those who, for physical, emotional or financial reasons, are prevented from having the one thing they most desire.

Gwen from County Kildare

After my first miscarriage, I believed the doctor when he said that I was young and could try again, and that I'd be pregnant in no time. I didn't think that the next time I'd see him would be sixteen months later, when I was having my second miscarriage. This time, he assured me it wouldn't take another thirteen months to conceive again. (He was right: it took me eighteen months.) I asked for help, and he said I didn't need any. I asked question after question, and eventually he ran out of answers: he couldn't – or wouldn't – help me.

It's a very lonely time after you lose a baby, and for me the medical profession had nothing to offer me. The doctors said to me that I would have another baby, but it's not like I dropped a vase and needed to replace it: I wanted the baby I was carrying. Medically, I felt that I was looked after while I miscarried, but emotionally, I was totally disregarded – there wasn't even a phone number I could ring for help. There was no counselling offered and no follow-up care, and I suffered from panic attacks for three years afterwards.

I always believed that the only thing that would 'cure me' was a baby, and I was right. Ten months ago, I gave birth to a beautiful baby girl. This time I went to a new hospital – no bad memories – and was treated very well. My entire pregnancy was a very anxious time for me, and I truly believe that anyone who has suffered a loss cannot enjoy any subsequent pregnancies.

Trying again

How soon you start trying to conceive again after a miscarriage is a personal decision. Some doctors will advise you to wait one or two cycles, whereas others will say it's OK to try again immediately. It all depends on your own circumstances, both physical and emotional. If you have had an early miscarriage and are eager to try again, there is not necessarily any reason to wait. However, you should monitor your cycle and look out for any unusual signs, such as bleeding or cramping, which might suggest that your body is still coming to terms with the miscarriage. If you have had a late miscarriage, your doctor will probably advise that you wait for at least one cycle, as your body has been through so much, and will take some time to recover.

You may feel more pressure to conceive than you did before, and may find it difficult to think about anything else. If your cycle fails, you may feel as though you are miscarrying all over again. It is really useful to have people to talk to during this time, especially ones who are going through the same process. *www.magicmum.com* and *www.rollercoaster.ie* have sections on their TTC boards for women who are trying to conceive again after miscarriage. All are feeling the same fear and desperation, yet they manage to keep their hopes up and inject a little humour into the conversations too. There are similar boards on most of the websites mentioned in Chapter 4.

Once you see those two lines again, you will feel elated, relieved and overwhelmed. And when you've calmed down, the fear will start to set in. This is completely normal. Anyone who has ever experienced a miscarriage will feel anxious when they become pregnant again. You will worry when you have a pain; then you will worry when it goes away. The once-dreaded morning sickness will become your best friend, as the stronger the symptoms, the more likely it is that the pregnancy is progressing normally. This is not a foolproof system, as some women continue to have symptoms after a pregnancy has stopped progressing, but it does provide many women with reassurance. Most of all, you should remember that there is a very good chance that your baby is OK, and only a very small chance that you will miscarry again.

Recent studies show that the chance of carrying a baby to term after one miscarriage is 80 percent, after two successive losses, 76 percent, and after three consecutive miscarriages, 57 percent. The risk stays at around this level until after five consecutive losses, when it starts to drop off.

If you are very anxious about your pregnancy, you should arrange an early scan to put your mind at rest. Most maternity hospitals can organise this for you at around eight weeks. If your hospital or obstetrician cannot provide this service, you can book a private scan at one of the private clinics or hospitals. At eight weeks, you should see a heartbeat, and the risk of miscarriage drops to less than 5 percent at that stage.

You may have spoken to your doctor about support medication for this pregnancy. Many doctors provide hormonal support, such as progesterone supplements and HCG shots, for the first trimester. If blood tests have shown your progesterone levels to be low, you will probably be advised to take supplements. There is much debate about the effectiveness of hormonal supplementation, but there is agreement that it doesn't do any harm, so, if nothing else, it can provide you with the reassurance that you are doing everything you can to support your pregnancy.

You may also be offered blood-thinning medication, as clotting is often a cause of miscarriage. Even if blood tests have not shown any clotting problems, you may still be offered Heparin injections and baby aspirin, as, again, they will not do you any harm in the short term.

You may need some extra attention and diversions to help you through those nail-biting first twelve weeks. There is great support on the Pregnant After Loss (PAL) board on *www.magicmum.com*. There are plenty of women in the same boat as you: you can attempt to keep each other sane while you wait out the first trimester.

Good luck!

A final word

As I write, I am six and a half months pregnant with my daughter, Anna. I am not pregnant because I know a lot about fertility. In fact, I find the opposite is usually true: those who know the most tend to be the ones who have had the biggest obstacles to overcome and, as a consequence, the least success. I am pregnant because I am one of the lucky ones, one of the winners of the fertility lottery. I'm not going to tell you that it is all worth it in the end, because we are not at the finishing line yet and nobody can give any guarantees that you or I will end our journeys with a baby.

What I will say is that it *can* happen, even against the greatest of odds. It doesn't mean that it *will* happen, but I do believe that the more informed you are, the greater your choices, and the greater your chances of success. It is up to you to decide how far you will go, how much you can take, and to what extent you are willing to move the goalposts along the way.

My greatest hope for the future of fertility treatment in Ireland lies not so much in the area of technology but in the area of access. Currently, IUI and IVF are not available on the public health service, and insurance companies do not consider infertility to be an illness or a medical condition, and therefore do not cover fertility treatments. I have spoken personally to Bertie Ahern about this; he has said that he will look into the situation. At the time of going to print, the Department of Health and Children has not been able to give me a timeframe for any proposed legislative changes regarding assisted-reproduction services, although I have been told that there are plans for a certain amount of fertility treatment to be made available on the public health service.

I wish each and every one of you the very best of luck in your TTC endeavours. I hope I have been of some help.

About the author

Fiona McPhillips is a freelance journalist and academic researcher. She is also infertile. Since giving birth to her son in 2003, she has had three rounds of Clomid, three IUIs and two IVFs, and has suffered six miscarriages. She has documented her struggles on her blog, The Waiting Game, which is available on her website, *www.makingbabies.ie*.

Acknowledgements

Thanks to Cathy McKone for encouraging me to write, to Sarah Traynor for getting me started, to Joanna Donnelly for support, encouragement and proofreading, to Seán and Peter at Liberties Press, to all those who gave personal accounts of their own stories, and to John for everything. Special thanks to my wonderful family and friends, the bloggers and readers, the Magic Mums and the Fertility Friends for helping me through the last three years.